bro

good call

on picking up this book

BROTHERS
BROTHERS
BROTHERS
BROTHERS
BROTHERS
BROTHERS

The *Real* Bro Code

The essential guide for dudes on
how to be a bro

by Kim Evensen

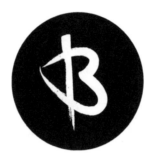

Published in Norway by Brothers. For worldwide distribution.
Cover design: Kim Evensen
Author photos: Magnus Løvrød
ISBN-13: 978-0-6484829-2-5
Available as paperback and e-book.

This title may be purchased in bulk for educational, business
or fund-raising use. For information, please e-mail
orders@wearebrothers.org

Kim is available to give keynote presentations and lead
workshops on the topic of male friendship for a variety of
different audiences. For booking, inquire by sending an
e-mail to contact@wearebrothers.org

www.wearebrothers.org - @wearebrothersorg

THE CONTENT OF THE REAL BRO CODE

The chapters are many, but they're short and sweet.

DISCLAIMER

Though Kim has gotten full permission to share the stories and the interviews he has had with people, the names of some people in this book have been changed to protect their privacy. Kim is not responsible for any actions you may take, or others' reactions, when applying what you learn from this book to your own life. Kim is not a professional psychologist or counselor, and though he offers coaching, he does not provide professional mental health advice or support.

PART ONE
INTRO

BROTHERS
BROTHERS
BROTHERS
BROTHERS
BROTHERS
BROTHERS

Bro, you've made a good choice. A *really* good one. I'm pumped that you've started reading The Real Bro Code. Trust me, your bros are gonna thank you for it.

Before we continue, I want you to know that The Real Bro Code is a book for every boy and man out there. It's for the guys who haven't read a single book voluntarily and the guys who read three books a week. It's for the sports jock, the gym junkie, the musician, the tradesman and the business-man. It's for the 15-year-old skater, the college student and for the recently married bloke.

It's for the popular dude and for the guy who struggles to fit in. It's for the guy who's got lots of mates (that's Australian for friends by the way...), and for the guy who feels like he doesn't have any. It's for the man who is longing for an even deeper connection with his bros and the one who doesn't think he needs to learn anything about friendship at all. It's especially for the guy who finds it hella uncomfortable to even pick up a book about men's friendships.

As guys, learning how to do friendship well is not some-thing we normally learn in school, and we're not really en-couraged to learn anything about it or talk about it in general either. The Real Bro Code is therefore most likely the first book most of you have ever read about male friendships - and that's pretty cool!

Now. Let me start by introducing myself. My name is Kim. I'm a dude (to those who haven't heard of a guy named Kim before). I was born in Norway and I've lived a few years in Australia. I'm also the founder and CEO of Brothers, a global organization dedicated to empowering boys' and men's friendships.

I founded Brothers in 2017 because I thought there ought to be an organization fighting for and advocating for guys' friendships. Why? Well, because our friendships are some of the most important relationships in our lives, and they deserve our attention and investment. I figured out quite early in the process though, that boys' and men's friendships have become a more or less stigmatized topic in Western society. I've encountered many guys finding the topic both awkward and confronting - and I totally get it. The prevailing wisdom among Western men seems to be: Love your brother, but by all means don't express it or talk about it too much.

The dudes I've encountered who are put off by hearing about Brothers quickly admit that it's actually a pretty cool concept and that "brotherhood is really important." Interestingly enough, a part of my job is to normalize guys' longing for true brotherhood. Just like it's important for girls to have girlfriends, guys need guy friends.

As the leader of Brothers, I do talks, run workshops and offer coaching - all on the topic of male friendship. So far we've worked with sports clubs, schools, government organizations, other organizations/charities, and different one-off events. We also communicate our message through our online platforms (mostly Instagram & Facebook), through books, campaigns, and by collaborating with individuals, researchers, not-for-profits, movements, and companies.

Though I originally had no plan on doing what I'm doing now, only thinking Brothers would be a side-project, I've now ended up spending most of my time trying to steer this ship. And though it's a massive challenge, and though I often find myself way in over my head, I love what I'm doing.

The Real Bro Code is a book packed with stories, inspiration, questions, information and guidance—backed up with research—that will set you up to develop deeper friendships with the guys you care about in your life. As I take you through a lot of chapters based on different topics, I'll give you some good advice, principles and values that you can choose to take on board. You'll also, most likely, get some new perspectives on this topic, as I'll challenge some of the stereotypical views we have of male bonding in Western culture. Some of you will find this quite confronting, and not only because the topic (friendship) in and of itself is something that hits really close to home, but because it might make you question a mindset that you've had for years. But again, if we're not challenged, we won't grow.

The most important part is at the end of every chapter, where I've written down a few questions for you to reflect on. The Real Bro Code is based on and completely dependent on you reflecting on and answering these questions. So I can't stress this enough - carry a pen while reading it and take your time to write down your answers. If you've got the e-book you can write down your reflections in a notebook or on your phone. Though some of the questions might feel or sound a bit similar, there's a reason why they're there. So remember to take your time.

After some of the questions, there might be some suggested actions to take or I'll invite you to come up with practical things you can do to implement what you've learned in the chapter. Whatever you learn has to be practiced for it to make a difference in your life.

If you do all this, this book will go from okay to exceptional.

My job is to invite you to reflect on what you otherwise wouldn't have, so that you can take actions that will strengthen and help you get more out of your friendships. With that being said, I believe that you'll get as much out of The Real Bro Code as you want to yourself - so we gotta work together on this.

One of the dilemmas when writing a book like this, is what if I accidentally send out signals to guys that their friendships aren't good enough - or signals like "guys suck at friendship, that's why I've written this book." I hope you know that isn't my heart or intention behind what I do. It's important to appreciate our friendships and where they're at, but not stop there. There's always more. There's more connection, adventure and depth than what we've experienced so far. Some say that close guy friendships are seldom and rare and that male friendships have been reduced to shallow hangouts—a workout buddy or a drinking partner. That might be true to some extent, but I'm ready to see that narrative change. It is in every boy's and man's DNA to develop close, wholesome friendships.

You won't figure out who you are in isolation. It's in your closest relationships that you find out who you are, what your role is, and also what your blind spots, fears and insecurities are, not to mention your dreams, goals and qualities. If you have a willingness to learn, this book will expand your perspective and mindset on men's friendships—and every bro (and every woman) in your life will benefit from it.

Enjoy it, bro!

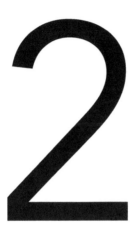

PART TWO
THE REAL BRO CODE

BROTHERS
BROTHERS
BROTHERS
BROTHERS
BROTHERS
BROTHERS

1: Brotherhood

Last night I was on the phone with one of my mates. For fifty minutes or so, we talked about everything. We talked about work, school, memories - we joked around and shared random stories with each other. Since we don't live in the same city, we started talking about seeing each other soon. Though we didn't have the deepest, most profound conversation, our conversation made me feel so uplifted, cared for and connected. Before we hung up, we both told each other that we missed each other and that we were looking forward to seeing each other again soon.

Before I went to bed, I really thought to myself: 'Wow... He's such a quality guy. I'm lucky to have him in my life." And I know that he thinks the same about me.

Brotherhood is important. Feeling like you belong and that you've got some boys to do life with. Not just someone that you reach out to once a month or call whenever you're in a crisis - but someone who's a part of your daily life, so to say. There's this saying I like to use: "If you're not present in your bro's life, then who is?" There are most likely some guys who are relying on you, whom you are important to. Just like someone is important to you.

Though brotherhood consists of many things, the core has to be, as cheesy as it may sound like, mutual love. We may play sports, chill out, have deep conversations, casual conversations, laugh together, cry together, all that. A brotherhood is a place to be accepted, loved and fought for. On good days and bad days.

I am forever grateful for my boys, and I want to do everything I can to become an even better brother. So I dedicate The Real Bro Code to them.

QUESTIONS TO REFLECT ON

1: Is friendship important to you? Explain your answer.

Yes, because friendship is family.
I don't have a close relationship
with my family so I rely more
on my friends for love & support.

2: Who are your best/closest guy friends? And why?

1 Kelly - We've been through everything
2 Joe My best man & took me in
during lonely holidays
3 Matt H - A quality friend & man
4 Colin - Calming force who gets me
5 Matt B - We've shared recovery

3: When big events happen in your life, or you receive really good or bad news, who'd be the first guy you'd call to share the news with? And why him?

Kelly, it's always been him
because he knows me better
than anyone beside Matt.

2: The Taboo

I initiated an interview with a young professional soccer player once about the topic of male friendship. I asked him why he said yes to being interviewed:

"Well," he said, "Because friendship is an important topic to me."

After a short pause, he added this to his answer: "But… It's kind of a taboo topic to talk about."

Before we had even really started the conversation, he had hit the nail on the head. The reality is that the topic of men's friendships, something that should be so normal to talk about, has become one of the most taboo topics in a man's life.

A few years back, I founded Brothers because I was sick of looking at millions of men missing out on real connection. I had seen how this taboo had created so much insecurity and awkwardness between boys and men. Something had to be done.

Brothers' goal is to equip men of all generations to have strong and authentic friendships. We also seek to combat damaging cultural mindsets that may hinder men from having worthwhile friendships in their lives. Though most people love our message, support it, and understand why we fight for it, I've heard some funny responses when telling people about Brothers:

- "What? Friendships between guys?" (followed by an awkward laughter.)

- "Wow, sounds a bit extreme to run an organization about that."

- "Oh, that's interesting… So is it a gay thing?"

- "A movement about guys' friendships … Well, is that really necessary?"

- "There must be something wrong with whoever came up with the idea of this whole Brothers thing…"

- "Please… Guys don't care about having deep friendships, especially not with other dudes. Girls do. Not guys. That's just weird…"

Little did I know that running Brothers would sometimes feel like walking on eggshells. People have so many perceptions about love, masculinity and male friendship. Post a photo of two guy friends and some people will think they're gay. Encourage guys to comfort each other when needed and people think we're trying to turn men into a cuddle club. Write an article about the overemphasis on romantic relationships, and how it may negatively affect guys' friendships, and some think we're against dating and romantic relationships. The list goes on. All the stigma and awkwardness around men's friendships is a clear sign that something has gone terribly wrong. And we need to do something about it.

Ask a five-year-old boy about his best friend. He will most likely gladly elaborate on him and his friendship. He will have no problem expressing his love for his friend. Ask a grown man and his response will be quite different.

Missing out on deep friendship is in and of itself sad enough. We are created for connection. Take it away and you'll remove one of the greatest gifts in life. But the absence of authentic friendship has tremendous detrimental effects on your mental, physical and emotional health, your professional career, family, marriage, and all your other relationships. Yes, it affects every sphere of your life, and believe it or not - it even affects how long you'll live. (Read more about the importance of male bonding on www.wearebrothers.org.)

Are you up for dealing with this taboo, once and for all? The more we talk about it, the less taboo it becomes. And though you might not think this is, or has been an issue in your life, you definitely know someone who is more or less affected by it.

QUESTIONS TO REFLECT ON

1: What was your first response when hearing about The Real Bro Code or the Brothers organization?

This is so badly needed but will it actually succeed in it's mission?

2: How do you find it talking about guys' friendships?

Awkward, uncomfortable, rewarding after the fact

3: How often do you find yourself thinking about your friendships? And what do you think about?

At least a couple of times a day. I think about memories & wonder what they are up to now.

4: To what degree do you think this taboo around male bonding has affected your guy friendships?

Destroyed some relationships

5: When was the last time you had a conversation about the topic of friendship with a bro or someone else? Write down what you talked about.

W/ Colin in the Mindful Manhood.

—

TAKE ACTION

1: If you're ready for it, share The Real Bro Code with some of your bros. Maybe you could read it simultaneously and discuss it with each other.

3: Deep Talk

Without exaggerating, every single guy I've talked to about friendship has agreed that when we dare to be vulnerable and share 'deep stuff' with each other, we'll get a stronger connection. And it's not really surprising. When you share something personal with someone else, you entrust them with information that they can, if they really want to, misuse. It's not really risky to talk about last night's soccer match or what you do for work. And though it's cool to talk about those things, we often want to go a little bit deeper with some people as well.

I once asked a 23-year-old named Zach if he could share with me one of the closest moments he has had with some of his mates:

> Definitely those times we've spent around campfires. Late night conversations. Moments when we've shared our hearts and stories.

Like Zach, I value those late-night conversations with my guys a lot. We don't always sit around a campfire, but you get the point. Moments when I share something, and then my bro shares something, and then we just end up getting closer.

Some of us find it a bit confronting to have serious or emotionally charged conversations with our bros - or anyone at all. I've encountered several guys who have expressed how it's almost impossible to stay serious without having to crack a joke at some point, when in a deep conversation. It somehow has to be humorous. If you're one of those guys, then I challenge you to not crack a joke next time you're having a deep conversation. Not because it's wrong to laugh, but because you daring to stay in the serious conversation might lead to even more openness and trust from your friend's side, therefore strengthening your brotherhood. There's plenty of time to laugh and crack jokes, so save it for a time when you're not using it just to avoid an uncomfortable moment.

Others don't talk about 'deep stuff' with their guy friends at all, and starting to do that now can feel overwhelming. You may not know where to start. Maybe you've tried to go a little bit deeper before, but faced rejection. Well, you're not alone. Let's have a look at Connor's story:

> One of my guys was hurt by a girl once. I could tell that he wanted to talk about it, but he didn't dare to. I know I could've changed the atmosphere. We as listeners often don't help in making the environment less tense and more warm and welcoming (for a bro to open up). If a bro has a problem, we don't make it easy for him because as much as he is trying to mask what he's feeling, we help him with it. We don't help him to get to that place of vulnerability. So we are equally guilty of it.

I could've been more appealing and supportive of my friend's pain. It is hard, though. I once tried to with one of my bros. I tried to make the environment warmer and give him the chance to spill his heart out. He just brushed it off and told me it was so gay. This made me develop some walls. So when bros give me hints that they are hurt, I don't always want to make a safe place for them, because of this one dude who described situations like that as being gay. I am afraid that they're gonna take it the way the last person took it. I'm guilty of that a lot of times. I pre-judge the situation based on my past failure instead of giving it a chance. [...] Without vulnerability there is no deep connection. Deep moments define a friendship.

Is his story relatable? Well, to me it is! And if deep moments define a friendship, then I don't want anything to stop me or my bros from having them. So if you'd like to take your friendships a little bit deeper and have a few more of these moments, then my advice to you is: be the first one to take initiative. Let a bro know that you'd like to go a bit deeper, or that you wanna share some of your story and your past. If that's too difficult, then show him The Real Bro Code, and it'll definitely start the conversation.

When that's said, remember that mutual disclosure is necessary to develop a solid and deep friendship. And it has to go both ways. A bro opening up to me is always an honor, and I don't take it for granted. Neither should you, or whoever you are opening up to.

It's good to remember that before sharing something deep with someone, we tend to evaluate whether we find the other person trustworthy or not. If we find the other person trustworthy, we might share something a little bit personal. Then, depending on how the other person responds, we'll decide if we want to share some more. So if you want to have deep conversations with your bro, then first show yourself trustworthy.

—

QUESTIONS TO REFLECT ON

1: How comfortable are you with having deep talks with your bros?

_____

_____

_____

_____

2: Choose a bro. How comfortable do you think he is with having deep talks with you?

_____

_____

_____

_____

3: When was the last time you shared something deep or some of your insecurities with a bro? Write down whom you shared with, what you shared, his reaction, and what you got out of it.

_____

_____

_____

_____

_____

4: When was the last time a bro shared something deep with you? What did he share? And how did you react?

_____

_____

_____

_____

5: Choose one of your friendships. Would you say that vulnerability goes both ways? Write down your reflections.

_____

_____

_____

_____

6: What can/has stopped you from being vulnerable in your guy friendships?

_____

_____

_____

_____

7: What's the best possible and worst possible reaction you can get from a bro when initiating a deep conversation?

_____

_____

_____

_____

8: Do you want more or fewer deep conversations in your friendships? Why?

_____

_____

_____

_____

9: Do you find it easier or harder to have a deep conversation with a girl/woman? Explain your answer.

_____

_____

—

TAKE ACTION

1: Initiate a deep conversation with a bro.

Tip: create a safe atmosphere for it to happen. A noisy bar, a party, or while hanging out with ten other guys might not be the best starting point for a deep conversation. Be curious about your bro's life and ask questions.

4: An Incorrect Narrative

Sometimes we accept a narrative or a view on something without questioning it or using common sense. We just believe that's the way things are. Here are some commonly believed myths about men and men's friendships:

- Men are not interested in close friendships with other men.

- Men aren't wired to be emotionally intimate with others.

- Men are only interested in sex.

- Men's friendships are more like "shoulder to shoulder" but women's friendships are more like "face to face."

- Men's friendships are about what we *do* together; women's friendships are about *being* together.

You might think some of those myths aren't myths at all. If that's you, I'd ask you to keep an open mind as we continue. To begin with, I want to suggest that emotional awareness and the desire for close friendship is a human quality, not a feminine one.

One excuse that many of us have gotten way too familiar with, is this one:

"Well! Boys will be boys!"

...And we use this phrase as an excuse not to change or take responsibility for our relationships with others.

Dr. Judy Y. Chu, author of *When Boys Become Boys*, did a research project with six young boys in the pre-kindergarten class at a primary school. She observed that when the boys "went crazy" and expressed typical boyish behavior, adults would often emphasize their actions. They'd say: "Look at him! Such a boy!" But when the same boys expressed what we often label as feminine qualities, like cuddling, being honest about their feelings, or when they cried or expressed admiration towards others, then the adults would tend to ignore their actions.

Dr. Chu once asked the dads of the young boys this question: "What are the qualities you love the most about your son?" Surprisingly, the dads mentioned their boys' vulnerability and emotional connectedness. The dads loved that their sons expressed so much joy, so much love and affection. What made it even more interesting was hearing that the dads also knew that most likely, these qualities would get tainted as their boys grew, simply because our culture expects something different from boys and men. How ironic is that! The qualities that the dads loved the most about their sons were the qualities they're later on in life being trained away from expressing!

I'm not saying that there is no difference between a boy and a girl or a man and a woman - there definitely is. But many people out there have wrongly labeled human qualities as exclusively feminine qualities.

Okay, so we've got some incorrect narratives of boys' behavior. Let's have a look at how this intertwines with boys' and men's friendships. You might have heard about this popular meme about male vs. female friendships:

Guy friendships:

Guy 1: Dude, you're an asshole.

Guy 2: Thanks, man. You're a bigger one.

They laugh together and their friendship lasts for life.

Women's friendships:

Woman 1: Girl, I love you so much! You mean so much to me!

Woman 2: I love you too! I don't know where I would've been without you.

They look into each other's eyes and hug each other. Their friendship lasts for six months.

Reading this, you might think "that's so true!" - but I don't think either of these caricatures are very helpful.

First of all, I'm not saying that jokingly calling a bro a silly word or teasing each other is bad. Many, including myself, have a tendency to be cheeky toward the ones we love, and that's fine. But. Words are powerful and we ought to be wise about what kind of words we're speaking to each other. A friendship where nearly all of the communication consists of calling each other insults or making fun of each other is probably a friendship that lacks both emotional intimacy and true, secure bonding.

If dropping the mask and getting real with each other never happens, depth is never created. And where there is no depth there is rarely any turbulence. No turbulence, and a friendship might last a lifetime (just like a car that never gets driven).

In a lot of female friendships, emotional intimacy and expression is accepted and even encouraged. That's a good thing, but again, that doesn't mean that their friendships are necessarily deep or solid. Words are cheap if our actions don't back them up. If we say, "I love you," we should also show it. I've encountered women showering their girlfriends with words of affirmation they don't really mean. In one moment they might cuddle - the next moment they will gossip about each other behind their friend's back. If that's the case, then yes – I understand why their friendship might last for only six months.

I've seen both women's and men's friendships last forever and I've also seen both last for a short season only. And there might be many reasons that determine a friendship's length. But I believe that if a friendship is deep enough, it will endure turbulence. What we do when we face conflicts is up to us. Do we fight for each other, or do we flee from each other?

My wish is for you to have both long-lasting and deep friendships. But remember that long-lasting friendships aren't necessarily healthy ones.

I've heard people say that "men's friendships are more like shoulder-to-shoulder friendships. We fight alongside each other, like warriors." Though it sounds cool, it may be harmful, because it forces men to behave in a certain way in their friendships, and anything else is considered unnatural or wrong.

It also pushes men into isolation and it ignores men's need and desire for closeness, one of the most important human qualities. I asked a dude what he wanted the most in a friendship, and his answer was, "I just want to be genuinely loved and cared for." That doesn't sound like a shoulder-to-shoulder friendship to me. It sounds like a face-to-face friendship, which I believe we're all created for.

Both men's and women's friendships involve looking at each other (face to face) and ahead and outwards (shoulder to shoulder). It's not either-or; it's both. And both are significant.

Some also say men are only interested in *doing* things together, and not in simply *being* together. That is the stupidest thing I've ever heard. If a man cannot connect with someone unless he's doing something, he needs to face his fear. A solid friendship has to be built on more than just common activities. If your friendship with your best bro is only built on your common interest in football, then what happens if one of you stop playing it? Remove football and it'll remove your friendship. Does that sound like a solid foundation?

Again, a child is fully able to connect and bond without 'doing things.' A child can look at you for ages and be mesmerized by just being with you. They're also able to bond through activities, whether by playing football, building sandcastles, wrestling, or playing a video game. They can do both, and both are important. So let's not limit men's capacity. Men are fully capable of connecting deeply with other people – some of us just need to relearn how to do it.

I once had a chat with Niobe Way. She's a professor of developmental psychology at New York University and the author of multiple books and hundreds of journal articles. She's done a top-notch TEDMED talk and she's been researching friendships among boys for years. She's someone I respect and I thank her for her research, wisdom and insight into male relationships. Anyway, as we were chatting about boys and friendship over the phone, she talked about the importance of normalizing boys' and men's desire and longing for friendship in a culture that doesn't allow them to. Popular culture might say that boys and men don't need or want friendship, that they are hardwired to just want casual hang-outs. But research and my experience as the founder of Brothers shows something different.

Niobe's research with teenage boys indicates that about 80% of them speak openly in their interviews about their deep affection and love for their best male friends. They even express deep sadness if in a conflict with a friend. She also told me about an occasion when she was discussing friend- ships with a classroom of twelve-year-old boys. After she read aloud a passage from her book (where one of the interviewed boys talks explicitly about his deep affection for his best friend), the boys in the classroom started giggling. Niobe knew exactly why, but she still asked why they were laughing. At first, none of the boys wanted to tell her, but after a little while, one of the boys said, "Well … because he sounds gay."

Of course, Niobe knew what the boys would answer, but she wanted them to put words to it themselves. And she took the chance to remind them that desiring close friendship – and even being hurt when facing trials in our friendships – is normal and good, and that it has nothing to do with our sex- uality but all to do with our humanity. She told them that most teenage boys sound like this over the course of adoles- cence. There was silence in the room… And then the boys started opening up about their longing for deep friendships.

What Niobe did here was normalize the boys' desire for connections with other boys. These boys had different per- sonalities, but they all had this in common.

What's cool is that I experienced the exact same thing as Niobe experienced (guys giggling when being introduced to the topic) when I had a talk about male bonding in front of over a hundred sixteen-year-old boys at a high school. I was not surprised, and I was well aware of the culture these boys had grown up in.

"What culture?" you may ask. Well. Here's an excerpt of the chapter "Superman Is Desperate For Friendship" from my first book:

> Think about all the entertainment we consume daily: TV shows, movies, music, ads – you name it. Take movies; describe the main male characters in most action and superhero movies. How do they behave, and what do they want? Do they have any close friendships? Are they loving or caring towards others, or do they appear as constantly strong, emotionally stoic and independent? Last time I watched a Superman movie, he wasn't really into friendships. He was a lone, strong wolf, trying to save the world and win the girl.
>
> I do like these kinds of movies; they're cool. A part of me would love to identify with the heroes in the movies; they make me feel like … a man. And I want to feel like a man, don't I? But let's be real. If I'd become friends with Superman, I don't think we'd have the best or the deepest friendship – it would take time for him to relearn how to be close to people. Superman might be cool, but he's not a good role model when it comes to building worthwhile relationships.
>
> What about other movies, such as comedies? In most comedies I've watched, the main character's friends

are mostly stupid or lazy or there to encourage him to get laid. Sometimes the male protagonist might have a friendship, but it's often just a series of shallow hang-outs.

So here's my point: if we let popular culture set the standards for our friendships, we won't attain many meaningful ones.

Okay. So basically, our narrative and conception of male friendship more or less needs a correction, all depending on how affected each one of us have been by the culture around us. And remember that I'm not trying to narrow down our perception of male friendship, telling guys that "now you have to behave like this or that." I'm trying to broaden our perspective of male bonding.

Some might still claim that guys aren't wired for close, male bonding, but may I suggest that whoever claims that isn't paying attention in class.

—

QUESTIONS TO REFLECT ON

1: With your own words, describe a stereotypical male friendship.

_____

_____

_____

_____

2: Now, describe the ultimate friendship a guy could ever have (aka bro-goals.) Compare this with your answer to question 1. Do they correspond?

_____

_____

_____

_____

3: Any of the 'myths' about guys' friendships/behaviour that has limited you or your friendships?

_____

_____

_____

_____

4: Identify ways you bond with your bros by doing an activity together. It can be sports, working out, doing a hobby together, etc.

_____

_____

_____

5: Identify ways you bond with your bros without doing a specific activity, but by simply being with each other.

_____

_____

_____

_____

—

TAKE ACTION

1: If you tend to bond with your boys through activity only, then try to catch up with some of them without necessarily doing a lot. Grab a coffee. Initiative a conversation. Try to just be together, without being preoccupied with an activity.

2: If you're the opposite, then invite a bro to do an activity. Try a new sport, go out on an adventure, come up with a creative project you could work on together, write some music together, or something else that you'd both enjoy.

5: Competition & Comparison

Sometimes I've let stuff like competition and comparison come between me and my boys. These things simply build up a wall between us and make it impossible for the friendship to grow.

I'm not talking about 'healthy competition' - competing for fun or messing around a little bit. I'm talking about when competition goes from fun to serious and serious to damaging. Who's the best-looking guy, who gets the most attention from the ladies, who's got the best body, career or house or car? Our culture is obsessed with these things. Be the best, be the coolest, be the hottest, be the strongest. The truth is that there will always be someone better, cooler, hotter, or stronger than you. Plus our view of any of those things is pretty subjective... Pursuing this just brings us down into a pit of depression and self-obsession. We all engage in comparisons sometimes, but if we're not aware of these thoughts and blindly feed them, they'll be like little foxes stealing the joy from our friendships. I don't want that. And I don't want that for you.

For me, talking about it has helped me deal with comparison in my friendships. It makes you highly vulnerable but

I've simply told my brother that I've compared myself to him or been jealous of him, and that I don't want to; because it sucks. It also makes me want to compete with him and that's not a friendship. When opening up about this, I allow my friend to see my insecurities, which again will make our friendship more intimate and stronger. And hey, chances are your friend also compares himself to you sometimes, and knowing that you tend to do the same can be a tremendous relief to him.

Earlier in my life, I often competed with guys over women. I found myself using women as a currency to prove to the guys that I was a man, and it felt even better if it made me look like 'more of a man' than them. Not only is this disrespectful to women, it's also far away from real friendship.

Let's stop wasting time on competing with our brothers – whatever we're competing over – and let's focus on loving each other. You are good enough as you are. You don't need to prove it, especially not to the men in your life you call your friends. Knowing how bad it makes me feel when I compare myself to others, I've decided that I'll do everything I can to make it harder for others to compare themselves to me. I want the boys in my life to feel better about themselves when they're with me, not the opposite.

A mate of mine told me that "friendship is not an audition room." It's not a place where you have to perform or prove yourself. I couldn't agree more. Leave the competition for the soccer field or the squash court. Otherwise, it'll just create distance between you and your mates.

QUESTIONS TO REFLECT ON

1: Have you ever compared yourself to a bro? With what? And did you do anything about it?

_____

_____

_____

_____

_____

2: Have you ever experienced competition in your guy friend-ships? Write down an example.

_____

_____

_____

_____

_____

3: In your own words, describe what competition might do to a friendship.

_____

_____

_____

_____

4: Do you think there are traits of competition or comparison in your friendships that ought to be dealt with? Write it down.

_____

_____

_____

_____

—

TAKE ACTION

1: If competition has been taking too much space in a friendship, then initiate a conversation with your bro about it. Ask what he thinks about it. Maybe share some of the info in The Real Bro Code with him.

2: If there's something specific you've compared yourself to a bro with, then try to share it with him.

6: Comfort Your Bro

Guys normally don't talk about this a lot. Many guys tend to find it challenging when they're in a situation where they need to comfort another bro - or the other way around. But why is it really so challenging to give or receive emotional support from another guy?

Many guys I've met tend to find it easier to approach a girl, rather than a bro, for comfort or emotional support, when needed. A few weeks back, a girl told me this:

> I've got many guy friends in my life and they've all got guy friends themselves. But somehow, they all come to me for comfort and to talk about stuff. I've asked them why, and they just say that they don't do that with their guy friends.

Interestingly enough, she's not the only girl who've told me this. And again, I'm sometimes one of those guys myself. When I struggle with things, or when I'm feeling down, I've often experienced that my female friends tend to handle my feelings better than my guy friends. And honestly, that's a bit sad. I'd love to be able to go to my bros when I'm down because I know that it's important and that it'll result in a stronger bond between us. And I want my boys to be able to come to me as well. I don't want them to suffer alone.

Sometimes, it's easier to share our feelings after the issue is over, but not always during the storm. There are a few reasons for that. The first reason is the mindset that we shouldn't express weakness towards others - especially not towards another man. Guys just don't do that. That's bullshit, of course, but that doesn't mean we don't wrestle with this mindset.

The second reason is because of the uncertainty of how a bro will react. Will he understand or will he reject me? If I reach out for emotional support, will it get awkward? Maybe he'll laugh and tell me to get laid or get drunk. And though there's a reason why some guys react like that (it might make them feel insecure or they're just not used to a bro expressing his needs for emotional support), facing rejection like this can often make it harder to risk opening up again.

As a side note, a bro who rejects another bro who's reaching out, is not automatically 'a bad bro'. The brotherhood might be good, but you can only be so close in a friendship without being able to be vulnerable and comfort one another when in need.

Softness, vulnerability and emotionality are at the core of our humanity. Both young girls and boys desire and need safety and closeness. It's not something we learn; it's something we are born with. And babies and children are pretty good at expressing their need for it. But we all know that if you don't practice a skill, you may lose it. So it is with our ability to give and receive comfort. Parents love to see their little boys connect with others and it's beautiful to see them generously give and receive affection. But somewhere along the way, boys are taught not to do this.

I recall a few times I've caught some of my guy friends crying. And these or often the guys who normally wouldn't express any softness at all. These moments are prime moments to get closer to each other if we want to. It's pretty nice and I wish we wouldn't hide it from each other.

On that note, I wonder where many men turn to for compassion, since many of them don't get it from their friends. I wonder how many men go to the club to get 'closeness'. They find a woman (or a guy for that matter), they hook up and end up in bed – and their desire for genuine connection conflates with their sexual desires, leading to a false comfort. I believe that if a man doesn't have a place to be warmly welcomed and embraced, he will get something *like it* somewhere else, whether it's sex, porn, drugs, alcohol – even career or fitness, for that matter.

I want to be a trustable guy. I want my boys to feel like they can come to me regardless if they're happy, sad, if they're crying, excited or pissed off. No masks, just them. I want them to feel like they can call me and come to me when they're down - not just during huge life disasters, but whenever.

When it comes to *giving* comfort, some dudes have a

tendency to believe that if a bro is not doing good, you should just give him some space and not ask him about what's wrong - just to make sure you're not forcing him to talk about it. I've got three responses to that. Firstly, many guys might want to talk about it, but they find it hard to open up. So as a bro, it's important to encourage your bro to open up. If your mate is struggling with being honest about the challenges he's going through, then there's almost zero chances that he'd open up without you taking the first initiative and inviting him to share.

Secondly, many guys automatically withdraw when facing difficulties. They've been taught that guys shouldn't seek comfort and they should deal with it themselves. So yes, it's true that these guys 'want space' and 'don't want to talk about it', but that doesn't mean that it's healthy. I've had to confront a bro once because he simply didn't know how to be honest about how he felt. He was scared of his own and other people's emotions and he would just shut down or get really angry if he was hurt, or if anything got too serious or emotionally charged. Being his brother, I chose to take that conversation with him. It wasn't easy, but it was necessary.

Thirdly, sometimes we do need space, and it's a legit need. But as men, let's be watchful and sensitive to our bro's feelings. If you're asking him if he's doing okay, and he says yes, but you know that he's not, then try asking again - and let him know that you wanna hear him out. Don't always take a no for an answer, but also learn to discern when you should, and when you should just let it go and give him space.

Also. Though it's nice to help your bro think of something else (when he's having a tough time) by inviting him out to do something or go for a run or workout for example, don't let that be the only go-to whenever your bro is feeling down. Yes, getting our mind off of negative thoughts or doing a physical activity can help, but if we always do that, and never actually talk about stuff or dare to sit down and express our feelings, then we'll miss out on some great moments of connection.

We all have good days and bad days. And it doesn't matter what kind of guy you are, you're gonna get a punch in the face one day, so make sure you've got someone to go to.

Sometimes we think that the strong, confident or funny guys never need help, and we refrain from asking how they're doing just because of that. But everyone needs someone to lean on. No one is made of steel.

One of Brothers' online campaigns, called #talkaboutit, communicates something that many recognize themselves in. That might explain why it is, as of right now, the most shared Brothers campaign ever. You can find it online, but since this is a book, I'll describe it:

Two guys hanging out at a pub.

Guy 1: "How are you doing?"

Guy 2: "Doin' good, man! Same old, same old!"

Guy 1 (thinking): *I hope he's being honest with me.*

Guy 2 (thinking): *I'm actually not doing alright, but I*

have no clue how to tell him...

Have you ever been in a situation like this before yourself? Either being guy 1 or guy 2? I certainly have. Here's what one guy commented on this post:

> Most of the time it's better not to tell anyone cuz they will just brush it aside with the same old "things will get better" and it'll make you feel worse.

I once asked Josh, a 17-year-old guy, how it would look like if he comforted a girl versus if he comforted a bro. He said that it would feel easier and more natural to comfort a girl:

> If she would be crying, I would just hug her and not necessarily say anything. I would just hug her. But if it would be a guy, and he'd be crying or feeling down. Well... It doesn't happen a lot, to be honest. But I guess I would just hug him. Maybe not as long as I'd hug a girl. With guys, I also have to find out how comfortable they are with being comforted. I don't want to hug him or put an arm around him if it gets awkward.

Everyone is different, but every guy needs a brother to lean on. But if we find it weird or awkward to comfort a bro, and if we have to walk on eggshells to figure out how to, then something's wrong. Some say that girls are complicated. But I feel like if this is the case, then us guys are pretty complicated as well.

Some believe that men shouldn't need to talk about

stuff. Here's what I heard a guy say in regards to that: "If a bro is feeling down, we don't talk. I just know - and then I do selfless acts towards him."

Well. Though I honor him for being aware of his bro's feelings and expressing selfless acts, I doubt that he always knows how his bro feels without talking about it. I certainly don't. Sometimes I can sense that something is wrong, and other times it's obvious, but I can't read someone else's mind. Using our words (talking about it and helping your bro to process something out loud), actions (buying your bro a coffee because he's had a rough day), touch (a hug or a hand on his shoulder) are all ways of communicating and expressing comfort. Don't limit yourself to only one of them.

I myself am getting more and more confident when giving or receiving emotional or physical comfort from a bro. It's a bit different though, because my guys know that I run an organization about guys' friendships, so it's kind of expected of me, almost. But I still have moments when I find it hard to call a bro when in a rough spot. But when I dare to, it often ends up becoming a really nice moment. And it's always worth taking the risk.

QUESTIONS TO REFLECT ON

1: What makes you vulnerable?

_____

_____

_____

_____

2: When was the last time you approached a bro for comfort? Why? And how did he respond?

_____

_____

_____

_____

3: When was the last time a bro approached you for comfort? Why? And how did you respond?

_____

_____

_____

_____

4: Do you want your bros to come to you for comfort? Justify your answer.

_____

_____

_____

_____

5: How would you comfort a girl friend versus a guy friend?

_____

_____

_____

_____

_____

6: How comfortable are you with approaching a bro for emotional or physical comfort?

_____

_____

_____

_____

7: Have you ever ended up not asking for comfort from your bro even when you really wanted to? Why?

_____

_____

_____

_____

8: Have you ever asked a bro if he's been okay, and he's said yes, but you knew that he was not? What did you do about it? Describe the situation.

_____

_____

_____

_____

_____

9: Imagine that you catch a bro crying. How would you want to comfort him? And how do you think he'd want to be comforted?

_____

_____

_____

_____

—

TAKE ACTION

1: Next time you're feeling low, reach out to a bro.

2: Talk to a bro about this chapter.

7: (Quality) Time

If we wanna get to know someone, we need to spend time with them, and I don't just mean playing video games. In this chapter I want to talk about the importance of spending quality time with our bros. Bro-time.

If you're not spending time with a bro, the friendship will never grow. You simply can't have a close, growing relationship with anyone without spending time together. You can't enjoy the ongoing depth and closeness of a relationship without any commitment. And even though it's totally possible to have a great friendship with someone you rarely stay in touch with, your closest friendships should definitely require some more commitment.

A side-note: quality time is good. But no matter how much time you spend together, if you're not being authentic, your friendship will always stay shallow. So keep that in mind.

Let's move on.

I'm a pretty outgoing dude, and I love hanging out with the boys and lots of people. Gathering the lads to go on a trip together is epic. It's chill, casual and fun. It feels nice to have a group of guys I can hang out with. A 'crew' almost. A great part of hanging out in groups is that you include more people and you get to see sides of each other that you otherwise wouldn't have seen.

On the other side, I've realized how important it is to spend enough one-on-one time with my mates as well. If we're only hanging out in a group, we'll never *really* get to know each other.

The thing is that groups don't require intimacy. You can hide in a group. You can hang out with lots of guys, without necessarily have a strong bond with any of them or having to share too much of yourself. You don't normally go super deep; you often tend to stay on the surface level. It's safe, so to say. But quality time makes you more vulnerable.

Some dudes might find it a bit uncomfortable to hang out with just one bro. Maybe you're not used to it, maybe you are. If you're not used to it, and you wanna start, then start today. You could invite a friend for a beer, a coffee, or you could go play a sport together. Quality time is key.

QUESTIONS TO REFLECT ON

1: Which of your bros do you spend the most amount of time with and why?

_____

_____

_____

_____

_____

2: Based on your answer to question 1, how much of the time you spend together is quality time versus group hangouts?

_____

_____

_____

_____

3: How comfortable are you with hanging out with a bro one-on-one?

_____

_____

_____

_____

_____

4: How comfortable are you with hanging out with a group of guys?

_____

_____

_____

_____

5: Why is quality time with a bro important to you? If it's not, justify your answer.

_____

_____

_____

_____

TAKE ACTION

1: If you'd like to spend more quality time with a bro, take the initiative to catch up with him. Text or call him now to see if he's keen.

2: If needed, decide how often you'd like to spend quality time with the most important guys in your life.

3: On the other side, if you only hang out with a bro one-on-one, and never hang out with him in group settings, then maybe initiate a group hangout together with some other people.

8: Commitment

Western culture has become quite an individualistic society. To say that we value independence is an understatement. We take selfies, we create our own universes on social media, we do everything to become successful or feel fulfilled - and we strive after self-realization. This self-obsession can, and has, in many scenarios, created more space between us. Instead of looking after each other, we desperately try to look after ourselves only, creating our own 'kingdoms' built on self-obsession and selfishness.

Any thriving relationship or friendship has to include, at times, putting the other person before yourself, even when you don't feel like it. There is no deep friendship without commitment.

Some people find it hard to commit to someone. They just like to come and go as they like. They don't like it when someone else is relying on them or when they've been put expectations on. Yes, everyone is responsible for their own life, but it's also true to say that as a close friend to someone, I have a responsibility to love and care for them. When I choose to call a dude one of my best friends (and enjoy all the benefits of a close friendship), I simultaneously give up some of my freedom, so to speak. And freedom is something that we value a lot. I don't have the energy, time or emotional capacity to have ten best mates. So when I say yes to some, I also say no to others. That's a fact. And honestly, I'd rather have a few close friends than lots of buddies. As a super social guy, I've often found myself in this trap. I've spread myself too thin and realized that I've actually had no one who's close.

I had a chat with Ryan, a 27-year-old Australian. He's a typical Aussie bloke, always up for adventures, such a daredevil, cheeky and full of energy - just a super cool dude. And also, not the kind of guy who would be open about his emotions and feelings. He said it himself.

I asked Ryan who his best friends were, and he quickly mentioned Jeff. This is what he said:

> Jeff and I have been good mates since 2014. What stood out to me, is when I went to Canada a few years ago, a lot of my mates dropped off the radar. But Jeff just kind of really stuck with me. He didn't know that I was coming back, but he was keeping that connection.

We chatted together for an hour, and I could tell that Ryan really valued his mate. He once said that Jeff was the brother he never really had. He was someone who knew a lot about him, someone he'd trust with information and stuff he wouldn't share with others.

A few years back, Ryan and his girlfriend moved up the

coast in Australia. But then Ryan's girlfriend broke up with him and he ended up alone in a city where he didn't really know anyone else - and it was close to his birthday. When he told Jeff about the breakup, Jeff said that he wouldn't let him be alone on his birthday, so he invited him to come down to Newcastle and stay with him and his girlfriend. When I heard this story, I was reminded again of how priceless loyalty and commitment is in a friendship. Ryan would sometimes laugh and say that:

> It's almost like Jeff and me have had more of a relationship than me and my ex.

By saying that, he was describing the commitment in their friendship and the strong bond they had together.

Reality is that without commitment, a friendship will at one point or another, fade away or end. It's like a plant — if you stop watering it, it'll wither. If Jeff or Ryan wouldn't have stayed in touch when Ryan moved to Canada, their friendship wouldn't have been what it is today. It would probably have faded away. Though they both had girlfriends at some point (went through different seasons of life), they made sure they looked after each other and stayed in touch.

We might call each other 'bros for life' and say to each other that 'we'll always be there for each other' - but time will test our words.

I believe that if a friendship doesn't survive the various seasons of life, it's because it wasn't strong enough to begin with, or we didn't want it enough. That might be difficult to swallow – let me explain: we can't blame our circumstances for our lack of commitment. A child does that – but we are not children anymore. We are men. So if we want a friendship to survive a season, we gotta come up with practical solutions for it go from strength to strength.

Have you ever experienced a friendship fade away? I have, and I've often heard that it's just a part of life. And yes, I do think that some friendships are meant to be for seasons. But let's not use that as an excuse for our lack of commitment.

To be honest, many of my own bros wouldn't have been in my life if we wouldn't have chosen to stay in touch regularly, and intentionally taken care of the relationship. It's often also easier to stay in touch when the friendship is new and exciting - or steward a friendship when you go to the same school or work at the same place or when you live next to each other. But what about when you move away from each other? What if you change schools or jobs? Then you'll suddenly have to put in more effort to see each other. Yes, we should appreciate the seasonal friendships and the friends we used to be super close to, but maybe not so close to anymore. But I don't want to end up at 50 years old, married and with kids, but with no bro that I've had for more than a couple of years.

What about when a friendship starts costing you more? When it's inconvenient to help out, be there for him, or meet up with each other? Recently, a bro told me that he had been given a great speaking opportunity at an event. When he told me the date, I realized that it was on my birthday. To me it didn't matter - I was stoked for him, but then he offered to cancel the talk since it was on my birthday. First of all, I felt really loved and honored that he even thought of it. Secondly, I told him that I would never want him to cancel an opportunity like that, and that I'd love to be there, listening to him speak on my birthday, just like any other day.

I was positively surprised when I saw how willing he was to go out of his way without me even wanting to or expecting him to. It also confronted me and forced me to ask myself if I'd do the same for him.

If you want a deep brotherhood you'll have to count the cost; ask yourself if you're willing to pay the price.

Will you stick to your bro through thick and thin? Will you forgive him when he hurts you or betrays you? Will you love him even during times when he's not very lovable, help him when it doesn't benefit you, brag about him even though you had that argument last weekend? Will you selflessly put your bro and his needs before your own, and be a bro even when it costs you greatly? These questions are tough, but they're powerful. The less selfish we are the better our friendships will be - and letting go of selfishness is something that we'll have to battle with for the rest of our lives. But it's a battle worth fighting.

I would say that one of the reasons why loneliness is such a big issue in our day and age is our individualistic worldview. We focus so much on the individual, and we forget community. We want deep friendships, but we don't want to give up any of our freedom or carry the responsibility it requires of us. Just like the guy who's afraid of committing himself to one girl and is pursuing one night stands instead, we can often find ourselves be pursuing 'one-night friends'.

Too many of us have gotten so used to low-risk, casual friendships only, that any friendship with just the smallest amount of commitment simply feels overwhelming. As soon as the word commitment gets mentioned, you run out of the door as fast as...well, really fast - simply because you've never allowed yourself to get used to it. What should've been normal (commitment in friendship), have become abnormal.

Travel alone and you'll go fast. Travel together and you'll go far. Do yourself a favor and refuse narcissism and the fear of commitment to rule in your life and friendships. It only leads to isolation.

QUESTIONS TO REFLECT ON

1: Sometimes it's easy to spread ourselves thin. By trying to become everyone's friend we can easily become no one's friend. Is this an issue in your life? If yes, what would you like to do about it?

_____

_____

_____

_____

2: How comfortable are you with commitment in friendships?

_____

_____

_____

_____

3: How committed/loyal are you to your closest bros?

_____

_____

_____

_____

_____

4: Describe a moment in your life that shows the commitment

you have for one of your bros.

_____

_____

_____

_____

5: Describe a moment in your life that shows the commitment a bro has for you. And how did this act of commitment make you feel?

_____

_____

_____

_____

6: How willing are you to put a bro's needs before your own? And describe a moment where you've done it.

_____

_____

_____

_____

7: How would your closest friendships look like without any commitment?

_____

_____

_____

_____

8: How do you know if a friendship is meant for life or for just a season?

_____

_____

_____

_____

—

TAKE ACTION

1: If you tend to spread yourself too thin, choose some people you want to invest more into. Make sure that you follow through.

2: If, in any of your bro-friendships, there is a great lack of commitment from your side or a strong sense of narcissism, let a bro know about it. Then let him know that you want to get better. Invite him to let you know when you might need a little reminder.

9: Integrity & Accountability

Show me your friends and I'll show you who you are. The people you have the closest and spend the most time with will affect your decisions, your habits, your development, your impact, and ultimately your life. The more time I spend with someone, the more I have to ask myself if the friendship is a good investment. If I catch up with a dude once a year, I normally don't pay too much attention to that question. If I'm hanging out with him every second day, it's definitely something I should think about.

It also goes the other way. Everything that I do affects the people around me, either positively or negatively. It's important to ask yourself if you wanna own that responsibility or ignore it. Ignoring it won't stop the consequences, though.

Here's an example: if my closest guy friends do drugs, it's more likely that I'll end up doing the same. Also, if I'm the kind of guy who treats women with disrespect, my attitude will color my friendships and my other relationships. And so on and so forth.

Simply said, a friendship that doesn't have integrity is not a healthy friendship; it's a breeding ground for stupidity and bad decision-making and behavior. Position yourself in an atmosphere of negativity and it won't take a lot of time until you start being negative yourself. Position yourself in an atmosphere where guys only brag about how many girls they've gotten in bed (locker room talk) and it won't take a lot of time until this language will color your words, then shape your mindset and then your actions.

I've experienced guys using locker-room talk as a way of bonding with each other. They use women to prove to the other guys that they're real men - a way to impress the other guys with their latest conquests. This is a clear sign of insecurity. At the bottom of it all is a guy who wants connection. He wants to be accepted by his mates. Be one of the boys. Unfortunately, he is trying to create a bond through the wrong means.

As people, we often have a lot of blind spots. That's why it's important to be able to confront one another when needed. A dude I talked to once told me this (when talking about his mate):

> Jeff is always honest with me. If I'm being a dickhead, he's not afraid of letting me know.

I like that. The fact that he wants and expects his mate to keep him accountable. I myself need my guys to let me know when I'm not going in the right direction. I would've probably been somewhere else in life if it wouldn't have been for them daring to initiate the tough conversations. Therefore, it's important to make sure you've got a couple of boys in your life who can correct you when needed. It'll make you better and it'll set you up for a win.

That doesn't mean that you should be open to everyone's criticism. Choose someone you trust to be able to speak into your life.

—

QUESTIONS TO REFLECT ON

1: Would you say that integrity is important to you? Explain why/why not.

_____

_____

_____

_____

2: Are you a good influence on your brothers? Explain why.

_____

_____

_____

_____

_____

3: Are your closest bros a good influence on you? Explain why.

_____

_____

_____

_____

4: Reflect on your closest friendships. Is there anything that you often do or talk about that you know isn't good for you or the ones around you? (If yes, then how can you change it, if you want to change it at all?)

_____

_____

_____

_____

—

TAKE ACTION

1: If there's an attitude that needs to be confronted in your friendships, then do it.

10: The Art of Listening

We all like it when people listen to us. When people give us their undivided attention and take their time to hear us out. Listening is an art, and being able to listen to someone who's struggling, for instance, might be much more helpful than giving them lots of advice.

When a bro comes to me and wants to talk, whether about random stuff or about something challenging he's been through, it's my task as his friend to listen. My ability to listen often determines where the conversation goes.

Have you ever tried to share something with a bro once, but experienced that he hasn't been present or listened? I have, and I normally don't end up sharing as much as I intended to in the beginning. But if a bro is good at listening, and responds well, I'll often share more.

QUESTIONS TO REFLECT ON

1: Would you call yourself a good listener? Explain why.

_____

_____

_____

_____

2: Do you think your bros would consider you as a good listener?

_____

_____

_____

_____

—

TAKE ACTION

1: Next time you're having a conversation with a bro, practice listening. Put your phone away, try to express with your body language and words that you're present and listening.

11: Masculinity

I wonder how much time we as men in Western culture spend (either consciously or unconsciously) on proving our manhood. We carefully choose our words and actions, making sure that we express nothing other than manliness.

In *Breaking the Male Code*, Robert Garfield writes about a set of behaviors that many men subscribe to. Though this 'code' isn't very much spoken about, it has a lot of power in the lives of men. The 'code' sounds like this:

- Don't express your emotions (other than anger, 'manly' emotions or excitement over sports).

- Be tough, rough, and strong.

- Don't express too much joy or admiration when hanging out with the boys. (This might be suspicious.)

- Remember to talk about sport and 'masculine' activities to reaffirm to yourself and the guys that you're a man.

- Be a womanizer – because real men can score whenever they want to.

- Be independent and in control.

And by all means, avoid expressing any of these things:

- sensitivity and warm emotions
- dependence on others
- loss of control
- any expression that could be considered feminine or gay.

As men go about our lives, we're under constant scrutiny by other men: follow the code. Don't do anything that makes other men suspicious of your masculinity or heterosexuality. And if you break this code, be ready for disaster. It can result in total abandonment by other men. And who wants that? I certainly don't. I want the guys in my life to respect me, to admire me, and to think that I'm a man. So I better just follow the 'code' then …

Doesn't this sound exhausting? Well, many guys are pretty good at playing this game. It has become second nature, the normal way of behaving. I've communicated with many dudes who believe that 'real men' shouldn't express emotions, cry, talk about deep stuff, or express affection or too much happiness when catching up with other dudes.

Though following the 'male code' will give you acceptance from some men, it'll rob you of true connection with others. No wonder so many women complain about their man's emotional unavailability. He's bound to the 'male code', and he's become terrified of his own and other people's emotions. He's been told since the day he was born that men shouldn't feel or express warmth, love or dependence on other people.

As a child, the little boy appreciated warmth, love and gentleness, but as he grew up, he was shamed away from it, feeling that it's 'wrong' for him to feel or express these emotions. In Niobe Way's book *Deep Secrets*, we follow a few guys as they enter adolescence. When I read Way's book, I observed that these guys get stuck in this limbo. One part of them wants and desires close, intimate friendships with their peers, but another part of them feels like they shouldn't want, desire or need that – because that's not manly. It was okay when they were kids, but not as men. Therefore, as these guys grew up, they started trading away their emotional sensitivity to be 'one of the boys'. By doing that they actually lost their ability to form worthwhile relationships. By trying to fit in, they missed out.

I've experienced this limbo myself, and I still am, to an extent. But I've promised myself that I will continue to fight against the 'male code', if I can call it that. I deserve better. And so do the people in my life.

I have often asked women if they feel like they need to 'prove their womanhood'. Most of the time I get a no. But when asking guys if they've ever felt like they need to prove their manhood, I mostly get a yes. I find that very interesting. Growing up, I've heard the phrase 'man up' many times (and I haven't really reflected on why; I've just accepted it). When I've wanted to cry, I've been told to get over it. When I've wanted closeness or comfort, I've been told to get laid or get a girlfriend. When I've wanted closer connections with my guys, I've received disapproval.

As a man, I've been exposed to so many messages on 'how to be a real man' – and they've all left me feeling like a failure. I've realized that I'm not measuring up to those standards of manhood, no matter how hard I try. A guy I talked to once put it like this: "The cultural expectations of a man are impossible to reach. If you try to reach them, you'll always find yourself falling short." Not only are you reaching for something impossible to reach, you're also trying to attain something that is damaging to you and those around you. And hey, if you've ever felt like you need to prove your manhood, then I've got good news for you: you don't need to prove anything. You simply are a man.

I find it interesting, though, how boys and men in one way are encouraged to treat women with respect and not look at them as objects, but on the other side, they're also expected to be constantly on the look for new women to conquer, to flirt, push the boundaries, and be promiscuous and sex-crazy. I've even met some women who've reacted when a guy is not drooling when a hot girl passes him on the street.

Straight men are expected to do so, and if they don't, then we become suspicious. "They're probably gay," we say - because 'a real man' should be crazy about hot girls. All the time. Above anything else. He shouldn't really be a 'nice guy'. Do you hear how messed up this is? And when the boys who've been taught this gather in one room, this attitude gets reinforced even more. Being promiscuous towards women and embracing locker-room talk is celebrated and expected but also confronted and hated. So either way, you can't win.

There's a reason why men are dominating the suicide statistics along with the statistics when it comes to rape, sexual assault, domestic violence, crime, and other types of violence. Some write it off by claiming that's the way men simply are. Well, that's a lot of bull. Men weren't created to hurt others. Men were created to use their strength to protect, help and serve. But when men are taught to shut up, suppress their emotions and humanity—all while being encouraged to be promiscuous as hell—no wonder people are getting hurt and women are being turned into objects.

A friend of mine once said that if men are healthy, our whole society will reap the benefit. But if men are broken, our whole society will suffer.

If you really want to be constantly tough, in control, independent or emotionally stoic, then go for it. And though you'll miss out on the depth of real friendship and connection with people, don't think that your behavior will only affect you.

And just to keep it all clear: masculinity and manhood are good things. And I'm not saying that qualities we often associate with masculinity, like strength, courage and adventure, for example, are bad qualities - on the contrary! Sometimes we have to express our weakness and there's power and strength in that. Other times we gotta be strong and stand firm, whether for ourselves or for others. But the 'male code', which binds us, limits us and destroys us, is not good.

I've seen that it has become a trend to use the phrase 'toxic masculinity' lately. Though I do understand why people use this expression, I'm careful not to use it too often myself, because if we're not aware, we can start to get a negative connotation of the word masculinity. Masculinity is great in all its ways, forms and expressions. And we need it. I am a firm believer in the importance of having a father and a mother, both the masculine and feminine influence on a child. And though a mother in many cultures is associated as the caretaker, and the father as the protector, at the end of the day, both are doing both things. You don't want a mother who doesn't protect her son, or a father who doesn't care for or comfort his daughter. In an attempt to feel like we're in control or know how things work, we can become black and white in our thinking, when things aren't as black and white as we'd like them to. They're grey.

I've had many chats with various people about what it means to be a man, and I've read books and articles and all that kind of stuff about manhood. What I've realized when talking to people, is that it's easy to choose either two extremes. Some people, in an attempt to confront the 'male code', create another box for men to fit into. Instead of being emotionally stoic, tough and independent, they expect all men to now talk about their feelings all time, cry every day - and hold hands while they do. The other extreme is people who are threatened by those confronting the 'male code', and they look at it as an attack on masculinity and men, believing that 'they' want to turn men into wimpy, passive mama's boys. As a result, they reject any suggestion of a more wholesome way of living as a man.

My point is this: every guy is different: different personality, interests, culture, physique, upbringing and all that. Whether you're a really emotional guy or not really emotional at all, you're not more or less of a man. Whether you're the top athlete at your college, or you suck at sports but you're the smartest kid in mathematics, you're not more or less of a man, or more or less valuable as a human being. Western perception of masculinity is extremely narrow-minded, and unfortunately, masculinity has been reduced down to a certain set of interests or physical abilities, when actually, masculinity is so much better and so much more.

Every guy (and girl) is created for deep relationships with other people, to care for, to love, and to be sensitive and aware of their own feelings and the feelings of others, regardless of culture, race, socioeconomic background, personality, upbringing, sexual preference - or whatever else.

Now. Let me finish with this: let us not, by any means, try to change a man into something he's not. But rather encourage him to be all that he is meant to be.

QUESTIONS TO REFLECT ON

1: Do you think the 'male code' has affected you? In what ways?

_____

_____

_____

_____

2: Have you ever felt like you've needed to either prove or defend your manhood? If yes, then in what ways?

_____

_____

_____

_____

3: How did you express your emotions when you were a child compared to how you express them now?

_____

_____

_____

_____

4: What kind of qualities do you think your bros are appreciating the most about a man?

_____

_____

_____

_____

5: What kind of qualities are you appreciating the most about a man?

_____

_____

_____

_____

6: How good are you with handling your own and other people's emotions?

_____

_____

_____

_____

7: How good do you think your best bros are with handling their own and other people's emotions?

_____

_____

_____

8: How comfortable are you with expressing things like sensitivity, warm emotions or vulnerability, when being with your bros?

_____

_____

_____

_____

9: Have you ever found yourself using women as a 'currency' in order to prove your manhood to other guys or yourself? If yes, then describe a situation.

_____

_____

_____

_____

TAKE ACTION

1: Initiate a conversation with a bro about this chapter.

2: If you know a bro who's scared of his own or other people's emotions, sensitivity or vulnerability, then talk to him about it. If you struggle with this yourself, then mention it to a bro and figure out how you can get better at it.

12: Why Veterans Miss War

A while back ago, I watched Sebastian Junger's TED talk about why veterans miss war. In his talk, he shares thoughts and insights that I otherwise wouldn't have thought about. The key question he asks is: "How can so many veterans possibly miss something as terrible as war?" Junger believes they miss brotherhood.

I used Junger's example in a talk I had on male friendship and the importance of it, in the Norwegian Armed Forces once. I found out that it was a pretty effective example to use when talking to soldiers.

Imagine a group of soldiers in combat in a foreign land. They're far away from home, they're far away from safety, and they know their lives are in constant danger. And what they see and experience is nothing less than traumatic.

They know that if they want to survive, they better stay together and help each other. There is no room for selfishness. Their physical bodies and their mental and emotional capacities are tested to the limit, and the nightmare they find themselves in somehow forces them to become closer. What they see is too heavy for them to bear on their own, and they seek closeness and comfort from those they are with.

It's quiet right now, but gunfire and bombs might go off in the next minute. And the only security you have is each other.

In a situation like that you couldn't care less about what's 'manly' and what's not. Leaning on your brother's shoulder would be the most natural thing to do. Pouring out your heart and tears to your brother would feel nothing less than necessary. You somehow realize what really matters and what doesn't.

And then the war is over. You go home to your family. Maybe you have a wife and kids. And you finally get back to your normal life. The scars that the war has given you should make you never want to go back - but still a part of you wants to. You miss the brotherhood.

What is going to force you to get closer to the people in your life when there's no danger around you? Suddenly, you don't need closeness like you used to. Or at least you don't have an excuse to need it.

According to Junger, many veterans end up missing the deep connection they experience during the war. Not having this deep connection anymore is a loss. And with loss comes grieving.

I've never been in a war myself, so I cannot possibly relate to those who have. But I do believe it can be easier to develop a strong brotherhood when in a crisis.

During a war, you have to trust others. You have to think about the other and even risk your life to make sure your friend can keep his. But after the war, the ones you've connected so deeply with might be gone or live far away. And your friends who haven't been in the war haven't experienced what you have - so will they ever understand you? Will they reach out to you when you need it? Will you ever be able to feel that strong connection again – knowing that someone's got your back? Knowing that someone would lay their life down for you?

It awakens something in me, writing about this stuff. And honestly, I don't think a brotherhood like that is impossible to obtain outside a war zone. It can be hard to find, but I don't think it's unobtainable.

QUESTIONS TO REFLECT ON

1: Have you ever been in a challenging situation or season that has been the catalyst for you and a bro to get even closer? If yes, explain the situation.

_____

_____

_____

_____

_____

—

TAKE ACTION

1: If you've enjoyed The Real Bro Code so far, feel free to take a photo of you and TRBC and post it on the Gram or Facebook. Tag @wearebrothersorg and we might repost it.

13: I Love You Bro, No Homo

As a guy, have you ever avoided closeness (either emotional or physical) in any of your friendships with other guys? Have you ever added a 'no homo' after expressing some form of affection or appreciation towards a guy friend?

If you have, you're in good company.

The problem is the sexualization of love. Consider this: we are constantly being bombarded with sexual messages. Music, movies, ads – you name it. And it affects the way we look at life, at love, at relationships. I like to ask guys what comes to their minds when I say words like 'intimacy' or 'closeness' or 'love'. Most of the time, they think sex. No wonder many male friendships lack intimacy! Our culture has reserved intimacy for sexual relationships only.

It's okay to be close to another guy when you're three years old. But not when you're older. Because that's gay, apparently. But if you're a woman, it's much more accepted. Picture two women looking into each other's eyes, smiling and giving each other a warm hug. Would you assume that their relationship would be sexual? Now picture two guys doing the same. What would you assume?

"Well, Kim. This just sounds like a cuddle club. And honestly, guys simply don't need close guy friendships. Guys just hang out. That's what we do. Shoulder-to-shoulder friendships. Not the whole face-to-face thing. Women do that. Not guys."

My mission is not to turn men's friendships into a cuddle club; we all express love in different ways. But if we think that closeness is only reserved for dating relationships, we're doing ourselves a huge disservice.

I once chatted to this guy about closeness. He said that he really wanted closeness, but he didn't have a girlfriend. I asked him, "Well, can't you get closeness from your guy friends?" He didn't think so.

Growing up, boys across the world are taught that what should have been normal (close, deep friendships with other boys) is gay. They've been taught that if they express too much love towards another bro, they're either gay or girlish. So instead, they avoid expressing any forms of love or affection completely, and add the 'no homo' phrase after everything that can be misunderstood.

The hyper-sexualization of love is detrimental to humanity, and if we don't confront it, it'll continue to ruin us and our relationships.

QUESTIONS TO REFLECT ON

1: When I say the words 'love' or 'intimacy', what comes to your mind?

_____

_____

_____

2: Have you ever used the phrase 'no homo' when expressing love towards a bro before? If yes, then why? If you've never used it, why do you think others do?

_____

_____

_____

_____

3: How comfortable are you with expressing love towards a bro?

_____

_____

_____

_____

4: How comfortable are you with expressing love towards a

girl?

_____

_____

_____

_____

5: How comfortable are you with *receiving* love and admiration from a bro?

_____

_____

_____

_____

6: Why do you think young boys/children have no issues with expressing love and admiration towards each other?

_____

_____

_____

7: Do you think our culture's sexualization of love makes it easier to develop close guy friendships? Explain your answer.

_____

_____

_____

_____

TAKE ACTION

1: Share this chapter with a bro.

2: If you find it hard to express love or receive love from a bro, then talk to him about it and say that you want to get better at it.

14: Bro-Awareness

How well do you know your bro? How much do you know about his past, his success, his failures? What makes him happy? What makes him sad? What are his insecurities?

In this chapter, I'm going to invite you to reflect on some of these questions. Maybe you'll figure out that you know more than you thought, or maybe you'll realize you know less about your bro than you thought. Either way, I think it'll be helpful. An important key to a good friendship is to be aware of the other person's personality, history, strengths, and also weaknesses. By being bro-aware, it's easier to communicate with each other and know how to meet the other bro's needs - because we all have different needs at different times in life. I might struggle with one thing, or find something really difficult to deal with, but my bro might find the same thing super easy to deal with. And the other way. Being bro-aware will help us to understand each other so that we'll know how to support each other through life's ups and downs.

I've had countless conversations with dudes about their friendships. I'm stoked that they all choose to share their thoughts and experiences with me. What I've observed is that guys who I normally wouldn't expect to be very aware or interested in their bro's feelings or story, are often very aware of their bro's feelings and story.

Whatever kind of guy you are - we've all been created with the ability to create deep bonds with people around us. And if you don't think you're really bro-aware, then I encourage you to practice this skill. You being aware of your bro and wanting to know him even more, shows your interest in him and in his life. In any relationship, being able to adjust our behavior, so that we can, in the best way possible, meet the other person where they're at, is a great skill to have.

—

QUESTIONS TO REFLECT ON

1: Choose a bro. What makes him happy? What makes him sad? What makes him irritated?

_____

_____

_____

_____

2: Choose a bro. Are you able to see it when he's not doing good? How does he normally act if he's having a rough day?

_____

_____

_____

_____

3: Choose a bro. Describe his personality (e.g., he is very rational, spontaneous, adventurous, sensitive/emotional, introvert, extrovert etc.)

_____

_____

_____

_____

4: Choose a bro. How much of his history do you know?

_____

_____

_____

_____

5: Choose a bro. What are some of his insecurities?

_____

_____

_____

6: Choose a bro. Who are some of the most important people in his life?

_____

_____

_____

_____

7: How bro-aware do you think your mates are of you?

_____

_____

_____

_____

—

TAKE ACTION

1: If you don't know a lot about your bro's history, initiate a chat where you get to know him better.

BONUS: A CHEEKY LITTLE BRO-QUIZ
HOW WELL DO YOU KNOW YOUR BRO?
(Choose a bro)

1: When's his birthday?

_____

2: Where was he born?

_____

3: How many uncles and aunties does he have?

_____

4: Write down the names of his closest family (mom, dad, and siblings.)

_____

5: His fav hobby/sport?

_____

6: His fav coffee?

_____

15: Don't Ditch Your Bro For A Girl

Have you ever been ditched by a bro for a girl before? Or have you ever ditched a bro for a girl yourself?

We live in a culture obsessed with romantic love. Finding 'the one' has become the goal of many lives. In most movies, music, and media, romantic relationships are valued and pursued at all costs. Friendship, on the other hand, has become more or less neglected. Let's have a look at friendship in some other cultures:

> Anthropologist Peter Nardi, who has conducted research on friendships among non-American men, notes the extent to which male friendships are formalized in many countries and provides the example of southern Ghana, where same-sex best friends go through a marriage ceremony similar to that performed for husband and wives. In Cameroon, adults pressure their children to find a best friend, much in the same way that American parents pressure their adult children to find a romantic partner. In China, at least until the late 1990s, and in other Eastern and

Middle Eastern countries, heterosexual men, especially those from rural areas, hold hands with their best friends and regularly rely on them for emotional support.*

Now imagine doing any of these things in a Western country. People would go nuts!

I'm not trying to say that we should all just start holding hands or have ceremonies for our friendships, but I think it's good for us to get some perspective. Reserving all forms of commitment, warmth and closeness for our romantic partner only, is a very Western way of thinking – and I've been guilty of it myself. However, Niobe Way writes that:

Stephanie Coontz, an historian ... blames the decline of social connectedness on our twentieth-century notions of romantic love in marriage where a partner is expected to fulfil all one's emotional and social needs.

She also adds that:

...only in the twentieth century (and early twenty-first century), under the influence of Freudianism, have we found ourselves increasingly 'suspicious' of same-sex relationships and focused exclusively on romantic partnerships. These patterns may indeed help to explain the patterns of loss in boys' friendships.*

---

*N Way, Deep Secrets: Boys' Friendships and the Crisis of Connection, Harvard University Press, Cambridge MA, 2011.

It's sad to see how friendships often are at the mercy of romantic relationships. I've heard lots of stories of guys losing their best friend when a girl has entered the picture. A dating relationship becomes the number one priority in life and all his friendships are replaced by a romantic partner. For many men, this relationship becomes their only source of closeness and warmth; and that is too much of a burden for his woman to carry alone. We need closeness from friends as well. When growing up, we all need female and male love - and our need for both doesn't stop as we grow older.

Life is unpredictable and seasons change. I want to get a girl myself one day, and hopefully start a family and all that. And though my friendships will change, they really don't have to suffer from this.

Here's a classic example: A guy gets a girlfriend. This means good-bye to his bros. After two years, his relationship with his girl ends. He then realizes that he's got no friends anymore, so he either desperately begs his bros to 'take him back' or he tries to find new friends or ends up as a loner. Truth is that he could've avoided all that if he wouldn't have ditched his bros in the first place. But done is done. It's awesome if he can come back to his bros if they're willing to take him back. But I hope he'll learn from his mistake. True friendships aren't a hop-on hop-off carousel. Don't use friendship as a cheap and worthless thing that you leave when you get a girl, but come back to if you lose her. You don't ditch what you value. You ditch what you don't care about.

Throughout the years I've heard too many guys talk

about being betrayed by their supposed best friend who ditched them for a girl. It's sad listening to them when they open up about it. Some of these guys have also expressed to me that they feel like it's unreasonable for them to expect anything from a best friend when he's dating, so they just settle with their friendship being neglected, and they don't really express how they feel about it either. That's sad. But also, if they don't talk to their bro about it, then they have to take part of the blame themselves for losing the connection. It's not just the guy with the girlfriend who is responsible for keeping up with the friendship - it's both's responsibility.

If my bro is getting a girl and I just leave him or don't adjust to his new life situation, then I should definitely not say that he's the one ditching me. Yes, don't ditch your bro for a girl. But don't ditch your bro when he starts dating either.

Getting a girlfriend will and should affect your time schedule. You need to invest in your new relationship, which naturally means less time to spend with your bros or doing other things. But on the other side, if your girlfriend gets a new bestie, then that will and should also affect your relationship. If a new person comes into her life and becomes important to her, then you'll have to dare to give away some of your time with your girl so that she can invest in her new friend.

When I get a girl, I have to do my part in stewarding my friendships and I trust that my boys will do theirs, making every effort to get to know her and cheer on our relationship. My bros should inspire me to be a better boyfriend, and my

girl should inspire me to be better bro. A good dating relationship should empower your friendships, and a good
friendship should empower your dating relationship. It's good
to grasp the one and not let go of the other.

—

QUESTIONS TO REFLECT ON

1: Have you ever ditched a bro when you've gotten a girlfriend? Why?

_____

_____

_____

_____

2: Based on your answer to the last question, did you talk
about it with your bro? If yes, then how did it go. If no, then
why not?

_____

_____

_____

_____

_____

3: Have you ever been ditched by a bro for a girl yourself? How did that make you feel?

_____

_____

_____

_____

_____

4: Based on your answer to the last question, did you talk about it with your bro? If yes, then how did it go. If no, then why not?

_____

_____

_____

_____

_____

5: Do you have an example of a friendship in your life that has continued to grow after one or both of you started dating? If yes, then why?

_____

_____

_____

_____

_____

6: If you have a girlfriend, do you encourage her to spend time with her own friends? If yes, then how?

_____
_____
_____
_____

7: If you're dating, how are you currently balancing spending time with your girl and spending time with your closest friends? Based on your answer, do you think you need to do any adjustments?

_____
_____
_____
_____

8: Are there any bros you've lost connection with (more or less) that you'd like to take up the connection with? Write down his/their names and how you're going to regain the connection.

_____
_____
_____
_____

TAKE ACTION

1: If you're dating, talk about the importance of friendships with your girlfriend.

2: If you've let go of a bro and you regret it, reach out to him and try to fix it. It's never too late.

3: If you're dating, do something that can strengthen the bond between your girlfriend and your bros.

4: If you feel left behind by a bro after he got a girl, then reach out to him and let him know. Talk about it.

5: If you're dating, ask your closest bros if they feel like you're good at prioritizing both them (your friendships) *and* your girl (your dating relationship).

16: Bros & Family

All kinds of dudes will be reading The Real Bro Code and every one of you will be in different seasons and life situations. Though I won't be focusing a lot on this topic throughout the book, I think it's beneficial to talk a little bit about how to juggle friendship and marriage/family life.

Whether you're a 15-year-old dude not thinking about family life at all yet, a 30-year-old single dad, or a 40-year-old married man with three kids, creating a family is a season most of us will enter into at some point. I'll write a little bit about it here and invite you, as a married or single dad, to reflect on a few things at the end. Though I should've written a separate edition of The Real Bro Code for dads, I've chosen to wait a little bit with that for now. Maybe until I become a dad myself…

I've encountered married couples, both living busy lives, where their friendships have grown stronger and stronger after they got together. I've also encountered married couples who've completely isolated themselves and their friendships have more or less faded away. Therefore, I encourage every married couple to sit down together and talk about how you can practically integrate your friendships into your family. By keeping investing in your friendships, you'll also invest in your marriage and family. If you think that isolating yourself with your family is going to benefit your wife and kids or yourself, think again. Stronger friendships contribute to a strong marriage and a stronger family. Yes. There are married men feeling lonely because they've got no bros in their lives. So don't shoot yourself in the foot.

Here are a few tips on how to keep your friendships alive and thriving when having a wife and kids:

- Do everything you can to facilitate and create a good connection between your wife and your bro. The last thing you want is for your best friend and wife to be enemies.

- If necessary, set aside specific days for friendship.

- Spend quality time with your bros. Keep in mind that if your wife is always in the same room as you and your bro when you're hanging out, you won't be able to create the same intimacy between you and your bro, as if you'd be spending time together alone.

- Trust is important. Yes, you're married to your wife, but what your bro shares with you in confidentiality, you don't just automatically share with your wife. If your bro knows that you're gonna share everything he says with her, then he will definitely not be as open as he would've been otherwise.

- Have an open house. Your wife's closest friends and your closest friends are welcome. Anytime. If your home doesn't feel like home to your best friend, he most likely won't come over.

- Don't reserve all your commitment, closeness and love for your spouse only. Reserve the sex for her, but don't think that she needs to be the only one for you to rely on for emotional and physical closeness.

- If you have children, invite your best bro(s) to be part of your kids' upbringing. You might not be as flexible anymore – but that's all right. Invite your bro to help out and to hang out with you and your kid(s). He'll become an uncle; how awesome is that?

- If you're a single dad: Being a single dad doesn't mean that you have to be lonely or bro-less. Don't be afraid of asking your bros to help you. Bros are family. If you made the mistake of ditching your bros when you got married, but now you want them back, then asking for forgiveness is the only way forward, or you have to look for new bros.

Need more ideas? Sit down with your mates and come up with some. Be creative.

Having close and committed friendships while being a dad/husband is not impossible at all. It's a choice, and it's yours.

QUESTIONS TO REFLECT ON

1: If you're married, how good are you currently at integrating your friendships in your family? Write down some examples.

_____

_____

_____

_____

2: If you're married, how can you make even more space for your friendships in your marriage/family life?

_____

_____

_____

_____

_____

3: To the dads. How often are you inviting your bros to help out or hang out with you and your kid(s)? Write down at least one specific example.

_____

_____

_____

_____

4: To the dads. How good of a relationship does your kid(s) have with your best bros? And how can you improve it even more?

_____

_____

_____

_____

—

TAKE ACTION

1: If you feel like you (and your wife's) friendships have been neglected after you got married, then initiate a conversation with your spouse about it and talk about how you can change it.

2: To the married/single dads: Have a chat with your bro where you tell him that you'd love for him to be even more involved in your kid's life. What an honor!

17: Encourage Your Bro

I wonder how many times I've wanted to give up on Brothers. Honestly, I feel like it's been every second day. Sometimes I don't see the results I wanna see and I let myself get discouraged by that. Sometimes I might get a negative comment by someone who doesn't understand why I'm doing what I do, and it can really steal my joy. It's weird how one negative comment can make you forget the fifty positive ones you got before it.

The last few weeks I've gone through some battles in my mind. I've asked myself questions like:

Am I making a difference with Brothers?

What if I fail?

What if I should've done something else?

Am I simply wasting my time and resources?

I guess we all face seasons in life where we doubt ourselves and what we do. And it's during these seasons that I've realized the power of encouragement. If it wouldn't have been for my own bros encouraging me, I would've given up on Brothers long time ago.

Matt, one of my best mates, is awesome at encouraging. Sometimes he encourages me with words and other times just being with him or chatting with him encourages me. His presence simply encourages me! Don't underestimate how your presence in a bro's life can truly and profoundly encourage him.

I see it as my responsibility to encourage my friends. I know how our own thoughts and the world around us can discourage us - and it's crucial that we've got someone who truly wants the best for us, sees the best in us, and reminds us who we are.

We can use our words to build each other up or tear each other down. And there's nothing I love more than hearing a brother tell me how much he loves me and believes in me.

If you find it difficult to do this, then start practicing. A clumsy and stuttering "I really care about you" or "nice haircut, bruh" or "proud of you, man" is all it takes.

And remember this: if you don't encourage your bro, then who will?

QUESTIONS TO REFLECT ON

1: Would you consider yourself as an encouraging bro? Explain your answer.

_____

_____

_____

_____

_____

2: Write down an encouragement you've given to a bro.

_____

_____

_____

_____

3: Write down an encouragement that you've received from a bro.

_____

_____

_____

_____

4: Pick one of your closest bros. What do you value the most about him? (e.g., qualities that he has.)

_____

_____

_____

_____

—

TAKE ACTION

1: Based on your answer to question 4, send a text message to your bro and let him know how much he means to you. Let him know what you value the most about him and/or your friendship.

2: Choose to intentionally encourage your bros more often. When you have good thoughts about a bro, let him know, don't keep it to yourself.

18: Long-Distance Brotherhood

Have you ever been in a long-distance dating relationship? It can be pretty tough! It's not as easy to stay in touch - you miss each other, and you have to be much more intentional to keep the connection.

Just like we can have long-distance dating relationships, we can also have long-distance friendships.

Some of you might have a best mate on the other side of the world. Spontaneously coming over one night to hang is not possible anymore, and maybe you find it hard to keep the emotional connection with someone when you don't see them a lot. Out of sight, out of mind, some say. And it's often true to me.

As a guy who's traveled a lot, I now find myself in a situation where some of my best mates live in different countries than me, even different continents. In these friendships we have had to talk about how we want to stay in touch - and how often, since we're not able to see each other physically too often. Thanks to technology, it's fully possible to stay in touch regularly, even though you don't live close to one another.

The number of long-distance friendships I find myself able to sustain and nourish is pretty limited. And though I've got hundreds of people I could've stayed in touch with regularly, I've chosen just a few. A long-distance friendship takes time, energy and it's expensive! But to me, if I really value the connection and my bro, it's more than worth it.

One of my mates I hadn't seen in almost three years. We used to live in the same city, but then we both moved away. At some point, we both admitted that we hadn't been very good at staying in touch, but that we wanted it to change. Now we've set aside a time each week to FaceTime or call. In addition to that, we text or call sporadically as well. Though we sometimes forget, we both have to make an effort. A few months back I traveled across a couple of continents to catch up with this guy. It was honestly one of the best times of our lives. Though we've had technology to stay in touch, there's nothing like seeing each other face to face. We had so much to catch up on, and it felt like our friendship was on steroids! We had so much fun, adventures, laughter, many super deep moments. I got to meet his family and his friends, and I completely fell in love with all of them.

One day I got the opportunity to give a copy of my first book to my bro's mom. I had written a short message in it with my signature, in her language. When she read it, she teared up and it was so nice. She told me how often and warmly his son had spoken about me, and how thankful she was knowing that her son had a bro who really looked after him. Yeah... That one almost got me tearing up myself!

Long-distance friendships can be challenging, but if you have one, there's probably a reason why you've made all the effort to keep the connection.

QUESTIONS TO REFLECT ON

1: Do you have a long-distance friendship? With whom and where does he live?

_____

_____

_____

2: Write down how you stay in touch and how often.

_____

_____

3: When was the last time you saw each other face-to-face? And how was it? (Describe what you did, for example.)

_____

_____

_____

_____

_____

4: Are there any ways you can get better at nourishing your long-distance friendship(s)?

_____

_____

_____

19: Conflict

I love you bro, but sometimes you
really piss me off...

Conflict in a close relationship is inevitable. If I'd never experience conflict in my closest friendships, I'd get a bit worried. It's either a sign of a lack of closeness or someone's not being honest enough.

I'm not saying that we should create conflict if there is none. It's definitely not worth pursuing! But my point is that experiencing conflict in a friendship (from time to time), isn't a bad sign. If you handle conflict well, solve it and forgive one another, it'll clear the air and probably create a stronger bond between you.

If I say or do something that hurts my friend, I hope he lets me know. It's only then we can solve it.

Sometimes I've found it hard to let a bro know that I've been hurt by him. I've kind of felt like guys shouldn't get hurt by their bros. It's okay to feel hurt by a girl or something, but not by another dude. But now that I've realized that it's normal, and should be normal, it's been easier to express it in my own friendships. I like to say that where there is an emotionally deep bond, it's just a question of time until someone gets hurt or a conflict takes place. When it happens, just talk about it if necessary, forgive each other and move on.

Asking for forgiveness can be hard sometimes though. We have to lay aside our pride in order to do that. I definitely can find it hard to ask for forgiveness sometimes, and to admit that I'm wrong, or that I've wronged my friend. But doing the right thing doesn't always feel the best, right there and then.

As we live, we've got to pick our battles. So it is with conflicts. Getting annoyed at silly things and creating conflicts out of that, is unwise. We've got to discern between what's worth bringing up versus what should just be ignored. Pick your battles wisely. Which ones are worth fighting and which ones aren't.

We'll always find annoying things or character flaws with every person we get close to - and reality is that some might never change. I honor the couples who've been married for decades, who have embraced their spouse's whole person, their good qualities and their imperfect qualities. Doing life together with people sharpens you, just like iron sharpens iron.

Here are two important things to remind yourself of if you find something annoying with a bro and he doesn't seem to change or want to change:

- You're not interested in him being perfect. You're interested in being his friend.

- It's easy to point out someone else's flaws and be blind to our own. Be thankful that your bros stick with you, even though you've got issues that might annoy the heck out of them.

—

QUESTIONS TO REFLECT ON

1: When was the last time you and one of your guy friends had a conflict? Over what, and how did you solve it?

_____

_____

_____

_____

2: When was the last time you felt hurt by a bro? Describe why, and did you talk to him about it?

_____

_____

_____

_____

3: Do you think a bro has been hurt by you without telling you about it? Would you like him to tell you about it? If yes, then why?

_____

_____

_____

_____

4: Is there any resentment in your life towards a bro that you should deal with?

_____

_____

_____

_____

5: How good are you at receiving constructive feedback from a bro? Do you tend to be open to it, or do you tend to put up a defense? Explain your answer.

_____

_____

_____

_____

TAKE ACTION

1: If there are any unresolved conflicts with any of your bros, meet up with them and deal with it.

20: I Love You, Bro (But I Only Tell You When I'm Drunk)

Have you ever been that guy or do you know a guy, who normally don't express too much affection towards their guy friends unless they're drunk?

> Duuuude. You know what? I love you!! So much… Like I don't know what I would have done without you! You're my man. My boyyyyyyy! BROS FOR LIFE!

…And the next day, it's either all forgotten or you don't really talk about it.

A man I know once agreed with me on actually meeting up with one of his guy friends, to talk about how much he valued their friendship. We thought it could be a good challenge for him. After a few weeks he told me he'd done it. And he was drunk while doing it. So I told him to do it again… without being drunk.

Another guy once told me that he didn't really talk about 'deep things' with his guy friends, because he didn't want his friendships to become 'too serious'. I then asked him: "Do you want close friends in your life?" He said yes. And then I asked him what makes a close friendship: "Well, I guess it's by opening up to each other. To really get to know each other."

Well... I don't have to say anything else...

After interviewing several guys, I've figured out that some of them normally don't talk about deep things in their friendships (though they say that they can if they want to) because they're afraid that it's gonna be all serious and no fun. But that's simply not the reality. A friendship consists of many things. It consists of serious times, fun times, adventurous times, beautiful times, challenging times... you name it. And by 'getting serious' when needed — and maybe a bit more often than what we feel is comfortable—doesn't mean that you'll have to be serious all the time.

Popular culture communicates that a man isn't really interested in close friendships. He's just interested in messing around and chilling out. That's what a man is. That's what's 'masculine'.

But why is it that many guys, when being drunk, can't help but shower their bros with love?

QUESTIONS TO REFLECT ON

1: Have you ever been that 'drunk guy' yourself? Or does this chapter remind you of someone?

_____

_____

_____

_____

2: Why do you think many dudes freely express adoration towards their bros when drunk, but not when they're sober?

_____

_____

_____

_____

21: Closest Moment

I've had guys come to me saying, "Me and my bro … We've got such a deep friendship. We've been friends for years. It's awesome. Just priceless." But when I ask them to give me a specific example of this closeness, they often turn quiet. They're not able to come up with anything.

I've also heard guys say, "I can always count on him! He'll always be there for me." It's nice hearing them say this so boldly, but often I find that lots of men *say* they can count on each other but rarely do. It's like having a car that you never use, so you never know if it's working.

You can shout from the mountaintop that you've got the closest friendship ever, but if the evidence doesn't back that up, it's simply wishful thinking.

That might be a hard pill to swallow, but the faster you acknowledge the reality, the better.

I'm not saying that guys who say that they've got a deep friendship, don't have it. I also understand that some guys might have had some really close moments, but they've not felt safe enough to share it with me. But I am saying that if you can't recall any specific examples of close moments in your male friendships, the chances are that you haven't had a lot of them.

The questions ahead are going to challenge you. Choose to let them help you, not discourage you.

—

QUESTIONS TO REFLECT ON

1: Choose a bro. What's the closest moment you've had together? And when was it?

_____

_____

_____

_____

2: Choose another bro. What's the closest moment you've had together? And when was it?

_____

_____

_____

_____

3: What have these close moments meant to you and your

friendships with each of these guys?

_____

_____

_____

_____

4: Do you want more close moments in the future? Explain why or why not.

_____

_____

_____

_____

—

TAKE ACTION

1: Whenever it's a good timing, remind a bro about a close moment you've had together, and let him know how much you valued it. (This can be a tough challenge for some of you!)

22: Expectations

I'd like to talk a little bit about expectations. We've all got expectations of one another and that's not necessarily a bad thing. Expectations can be unhealthy if you use them as a high bar for your friends to reach and ditch them if they don't. We all need to be gracious and forgiving, and too high expectations are no good. On the other hand, saying that you have *no* expectations of a bro might sound really selfless and honorable, but don't use this as a defense mechanism to avoid being disappointed or hurt. If I have no expectations of my best bro, I have no reason to feel hurt if he betrays me, for instance. Or what if I end up in the hospital and my best guy never visits or calls me? If I have no expectations, then I've got nothing to say or no reason to feel disappointed or hurt — because I've got no expectations.

Some guys really dislike being put expectations on because they're afraid of failing or disappointing. These guys can't handle any expectations from anyone without feeling overwhelmed. And that's not good. But again, the other extreme is not exactly good either - having too high expectations and getting hurt or disappointed by everything and nothing. You know yourself and what your tendencies are.

None of us are perfect and we shouldn't expect others to be. That being said, healthy expectations are important. When the time is right, it's helpful to share those expectations with each other.

Have you ever looked at a guy as your best bro but then found out he looks at you as just another buddy? It sounds a bit funny, but a situation like that could've been avoided by talking about your expectations of one another. Communication is so underrated. We can't read minds, so it's good to be honest and initiate sincere conversations. Sometimes you'll have different expectations of a friendship than your friend does. If you don't talk about it and agree on what expectations you'd like to have in common, someone will get burned.

Since a 'friendship' or a 'friend' can mean so many things, the expectations aren't that obvious. We have to ask ourselves questions like: What kind of friendship is this? Are we just acquaintances, friends, close friends, or best friends? And what does it look like to be best bros and do we have the same perception of what it means to be best bros?

I myself tend to use the word 'friend' quite often. I might call a guy a friend or a bro, but that doesn't give us any insight to what kind of friend he is to me, or what kind of expectations I have of the friendship (unless I give you more information).

If you feel like it's necessary or it'd be helpful, openly talking about your expectations with your bro will set you up for a win. You'll figure out if you're on the same page.

QUESTIONS TO REFLECT ON

1: Have you ever talked to a bro about your expectations of each other and the friendship? If not, why not? If yes, describe what you talked about.

_____

_____

_____

_____

2: Choose a bro. What expectations do you have of your friendship and of him as a bro?

_____

_____

_____

_____

_____

3: Choose a bro. What expectations do you think he has of your friendship and of you as his bro?

_____

_____

_____

_____

4: Have you ever looked at a guy as your best bro but then found out he looks at you as just another buddy? What did you do about it?

_____

_____

_____

_____

5: Has another guy looked at you as his best bro but you've just looked at him as just another buddy? What did you do about it?

_____

_____

_____

_____

—

TAKE ACTION

1: If you haven't talked about your expectations with one of your bros before, initiate a conversation with him about it. Especially if you feel like you've got quite different expectations of your friendship.

23: Needy?

In any close relationship, relying on each other for support is not needy. I want you to remember that. Too many men think that asking for help makes someone needy when actually, the ability to ask for help is a necessity in any thriving relationship. If a close friend of mine asks me to be there for him if he's in trouble, I don't see that as needy or demanding. I don't say, "Dude, don't put that expectation on me!" I see it as a declaration of trust. Some of us guys put our walls up when someone asks for help because we don't want to be told what to do. The people we care about should be able to ask us for support without us getting stubborn.

I once talked to a 24-year-old American fireman about this topic. This is what he told me:

> Male friendships are hard. I grew up with only sisters. You kind of see that with girls, it's okay to be emotional, and to state what your needs are. But for guys it's like: "don't be emotional." For example if I've been feeling lonely, it doesn't feel okay to let a brother know - and then ask if we can spend some more time together. Or to say to a bro: "Hey, I feel like I've been hitting you up a lot, but I'd love for you

> to start hitting me up. If only one person is doing all the work, then it's hard." (...) These things are hard to talk about, because you don't wanna come off as needy or...weird.

When he shared this, I knew straight away that I had to add it in The Real Bro Code. I've totally felt the same way. It almost feels unreasonable for me to state my needs to a bro or let him know how I feel about our friendship.

The same dude also told me this:

> I'm the kind of guy who likes to feel needed by someone. But with my bros, it just feels too weird to share that I want to be needed by them. It's kind of not what guys are supposed to share. (...) It's just like friendship in general. It's cool, you know. But talking about our friendships. That's a no-go.

What a guy! So honest! Who doesn't like to be needed? I certainly do, and it feels really nice when my bros come to me or express their need for me, so to say.

Let me finish with this. A really close girl friend of mine, Natalie, came to me and told me that she really wanted to cry and just be in someone's arms for a while. She was feeling so tired and at the end of her rope. It was so nice because she was so honest about how she felt and what she needed. I invited her to sit down next to me and then I just put an arm around her and she started crying. For 30 minutes or so I was just sitting next to her, a lot of the time with my arm around her. It meant the world to her and I didn't really do a lot, I didn't even talk. I was just with her. And what made it so easy for me to help her? Well, she communicated so clearly *how* she felt and *what* she needed. And who am I not to put an arm around her, if I know that's what's gonna make her feel better?

Comforting Natalie made me think about how difficult it would be for me to express my needs so bluntly to one of my guy friends. Open communication should not be something reserved for women only or for guys to do only in dating relationships. To talk about our relationship with a bro in a good and healthy way is important. Note, though, that there are two extremes. Where one is being commanding, demanding, *actually* needy, and not really respecting the other person's boundaries - and where the other one is not expressing our needs or talking about the relational challenges in a friendship at all. We need the balance.

—

QUESTIONS TO REFLECT ON

1: How honest are you with stating your needs to your bros? And when was the last time you did it?

_____

_____

_____

_____

2: Why do you think it's normally more okay for girls to be honest about their needs, but not for us guys? Do you think it's reasonable for it to be like this?

_____

_____

_____

_____

3: How would you react if a bro came to you, expressing his feelings and his needs so honestly, like the way my friend Natalie did to me?

_____

_____

_____

_____

_____

4: Would you like your bros to be completely honest with how they feel and what they need from you?

_____

_____

_____

_____

5: How comfortable are you with talking to a bro about things you find challenging in your friendship?

_____

_____

_____

_____

6: When was the last time you talked to a bro about things you found challenging in your friendship?

_____

_____

_____

_____

7: Have you ever avoided expressing your needs to a brother? Why?

_____

_____

_____

_____

TAKE ACTION

1: Next time you're in need, let a bro know.

2: Talk to a bro about this chapter and the questions.

24: Don't Ditch Your Bro. Ditch Your Phone

A while back, Brothers posted a video campaign on social media called "Don't ditch your bro. Ditch your phone." The message of the campaign was simple: Don't be so bound by your phone that you're not present with your bro.

It's a 21st-century issue. The new drug. Our phones. They're so helpful, but without boundaries they can be quite destructive. And it gets even more isolating when we've got our AirPods in our ears constantly.

I've often found myself checking my phone once every five minutes for no reason. It's like it's become a habit, and I just automatically do it. It's a bad enough habit to have when I'm alone, and it's even worse when I'm hanging out with a bro.

I've sometimes been told off by my bros because I've been on my phone too much - and I haven't always taken it well. Sometimes I've gone into self-defense mode and told them to care about their own business instead.

The thing is that if I'm in a friendship with someone,

everything I do affects the other person.

If I'm sitting on my phone all night while hanging out with a bro, what kind of signals am I sending to him and to the ones around me? I'm actually communicating that I'm more interested in what's on my screen than in him.

I've heard people say that you can be on your phone while being present. Well... For the sake of the argument, let's say that you can, then. I might believe that I can be on my phone all night and still claim I'm being present, but that doesn't mean that my bro feels that I'm being present with him. It's not so much about what I feel; it's about what my bro feels.

Technology has also affected the way we communicate. Most of the time it's good, but it has also brought some challenges with it. If we only express ourselves or our feelings through texting or messaging, for example, then we'll suddenly not be able to do it face-to-face anymore. I know of people who are super uncomfortable with talking about how they feel or solve inter-relational conflicts when they're face-to-face, but they're fully capable of it when texting.

Technology is supposed to be a tool, not a substitute for face-to-face communication. If we're not intentional about how and how often we use our phones, they'll destroy the intimacy between you and your friends and your other relationships.

Whatever you're able to withstand from you're free from. Let's be free from our phone, not bound by it.

QUESTIONS TO REFLECT ON

1: Do you think you might be using your phone too much when with your bros?

_____

_____

_____

_____

2: Can you think of a situation where you've tried to connect, but hasn't been able to because technology was distracting you?

_____

_____

_____

_____

3: Do you tend to talk about 'real stuff' in person or via text messages/phone calls? Explain why.

_____

_____

_____

_____

TAKE ACTION

1: If you think it's needed, write down a few practical steps you can take to use your phone less when being with your bros.

_____

_____

_____

_____

25: Ditch the Cool Pose

If I spend my whole life trying to act 'cool' around my bros,
they will never actually know me for who I am.

Too many guys are playing this game. Putting up a cool facade around their mates, trying to impress, trying to make
themselves look better in front of others, laughing when another guy says or does something not so cool, and by all
means trying to avoid being that guy themselves. What is
supposed to be a place of authentic brotherhood has become an audition room. And they're not getting out of it.

The truth is that insecurity makes us do that. If we're not
sure people are going to accept or love us for who we are, it's
easy to put up a facade. By doing that, we avoid being vulnerable by convincing ourselves that if someone rejects us,
it's only the fake persona—the pose—that they are rejecting.

You might not find this being an issue in your friendships, but if you do, then my encouragement to you is to do
something about it. You can spend time with your bro every
day, but unless you're being fully authentic and fully vulnerable, your friendship will never be strong enough.

I once asked Lubanzi, a 23-year-old South African dude, if he had found any challenges with getting close in his guy friendships. Here's his answer:

> Quite a few challenges, actually. The biggest challenge is that we're not really authentic. We just talk about sports, cars, how good Liverpool is doing in the league. And we talk about chicks. Most of the stuff that we talk about is about our accomplishments. It's all materialistic in some way. There's really no personal, close connection where we get to talk about our struggles. We all try to mask our lives with this outward persona of 'everything is going good' and 'nothing has changed'. We're so closed up, trying to hide our fears and failures.

Lubanzi noted that though he found this being a big challenge in most of his guy friendships, it wasn't an issue at all with his best bro, Bandile. They had gotten past that cool pose, and they trusted each other fully - and as a result, the connection between them was real deep.

We live in a time where posting half-naked photos of ourselves on Instagram, for the whole world to see - is fine, but exposing our heart to our closest ones is not.

Instead of spending all your time and energy on keeping a cool facade (which doesn't help you anyway), choose to risk living without it. Ditch the cool pose once and for all and let authenticity permeate everything that you do and every friendship that you have.

QUESTIONS TO REFLECT ON

1: Have you ever experienced any of your guy friends putting on a 'cool mask' or another form of facade when being with you? If yes, then what do you think is the reason behind it?

_____

_____

_____

_____

2: Have you ever put on a 'cool mask' in your guy friend-ships? If yes, then why?

_____

_____

_____

_____

3: Why is authenticity in a brotherhood important?

_____

_____

_____

_____

TAKE ACTION

1: If you feel like there is a lack of authenticity in some of your brotherhoods, initiate a conversation and talk about it. Even if it's you who sometimes tries to impress or act cool yourself.

26: We Need Adventure

Last year I went on a two-day hiking trip with one of my mates. We hired a cabriolet (the best decision) and drove into the countryside of Norway—beautiful nature that just wows you. We brought a tent, sleeping bags, food, warm clothes, lots of water, a little bit of beer, and all the stuff you bring for a night out in the woods. None of us has really grown up 'in the wild', so we laughed and said that we hoped we'd survive the trip. It was a test to see if we were real wilderness guys.

It was such a good trip. Hiking for hours in the middle of nowhere with a view that I don't know how to describe in a book. Sleeping outside in nature, bonfires, good company, lots of laughter and good conversations. It's self-explanatory that we had a good time and that we really bonded during that trip.

There's something about going on adventures together, being outside in nature, that really facilitates a space for good connection. Doing something you might not be so used to, getting a break from everyday life and the distractions of technology, having to work together and look after each other. Going on a trip and exploring and experiencing something together brought us closer to each other as brothers.

Since it was just the two of us, we had no chance to hide, which we could've done in a group. We were forced to just be ourselves, without masks. Sitting around the bonfire, having deep conversations, and then, for a little while, sitting there without saying a word, just looking into the flames. It was awesome. It's good to be able to be completely silent in each other's company as well.

Day two involved us hiking back to the car, jumping into an ice-cold lake since we didn't have any showers, exploring and climbing to a mountain top, and then drive back home to the city. We were like two super stoked kids both before, during and after the trip.

Adventure is important. A life without adventure will make you lose your drive and passion for life. Whatever kinds of adventures you like to go on, they get ten times better when doing them with a bro or some bros.

My mate and I still look back at our trip, and we often find ourselves talking about the memories we created together. Epic.

QUESTIONS TO REFLECT ON

1: Write down a cool adventure you've been on with a bro/ your bros. Who did you go with?

_____

_____

_____

_____

_____

2: Based on your answer above, how did you bond with your bro(s) during this adventure?

_____

_____

_____

_____

_____

3: What's an adventure that's on your bucket list of things to do?

_____

_____

_____

_____

TAKE ACTION

1: Plan a cool adventure and invite one or more of your bros to join.

27: Passive or Intentional?

Have you ever met a dude who once used to be full of life and adventure, but after a while, started becoming... kind of boring?

He used to care about the people around him, but now he rarely cares about what happens around him at all. He used to have dreams and aspirations, but now it seems like he lacks purpose. He once took responsibility for his life, his job, and his relationships, but now, these areas of his life have slowly withered as a result of his neglect. Reading this, you might think of someone who fits this description. But hey, let's be real. This might have been you at some point in life as well.

Here's the thing: I don't want to be a passive man. I want to be a man who lives with a purpose. A man who takes responsibility over his life. One of the friendship values we have in Brothers is this: "A man needs brothers that can challenge him to become a better man—a man who takes responsibility in every sphere of life."

I have met men who take a lot of responsibility when it comes to certain things, but they take little or no responsibility for other things. Here's an example: A guy works out every day to make sure that his body stays in shape, but he is completely passive in his relationship with his girlfriend. Another example is: A guy is all-in and responsible and intentional in his relationship with his girlfriend, but he is completely passive in his friendships.

According to Google (gotta love Google), passive simply means 'accepting or allowing what happens or what others do, without active response or resistance'. So with that in mind, I definitely don't want to have a passive attitude towards things in my life that are important — especially my friendships.

Okay, so what can passiveness look like in friendships? Let me do some brainstorming:

- You rarely meet up with your friends.

- You do make new friends, but you lose them quickly (friendships always simply tend to fade away).

- You never have time to be with your friends.

- You rarely or never reach out to your friends or take the initiative to spend time together. It goes the other way around.

- You don't really care about the depth of your friendships.

Passiveness can look like lots of things, but there you got a few examples.

An excuse I hear too often is: "I don't have time to be with my bros… I'm too busy at the moment." My response to that excuse is this: you make time for what you value the most. And the truth is that you'll always be 'busy' in life somehow. If you're not studying, you'll be working, if you're not working, you'll most likely one day have a family to take care of, if you don't have a family to take care of, you'll have projects to do, if you don't have projects to do, there's probably something else to do. And the list goes on. If you don't make time for your closest friendships, you simply don't value them enough.

I think it's important to reflect on our friendships and ask ourselves: am I passive or intentional? By the way, being intentional doesn't mean you're not letting the friendship be organic. I think there are times when we should just 'take it as it comes' and times when we should be more intentional. Let's be intentional with being authentic and honest and loving. But don't try to control a friendship, forcing it to look a specific way.

I remember one of my best bros and how we first met. I would have never guessed that he'd become one of my best bros back then (many years ago), but he did. We weren't trying to 'make a friendship' — it just happened. We were just being ourselves, letting the other person know who we were. It resulted in one of the deepest friendships I've ever had and it'd break my heart if I'd lose him.

A friendship goes through different seasons and sometimes we need to be a bit more intentional than other times.

That doesn't mean we won't have to compromise a bit, embrace change or be patient and gracious towards each other. But it means that the friendship can continue to grow not just in one season, but through them all.

—

QUESTIONS TO REFLECT ON

1: Would you consider yourself passive in your friendships? If yes, then describe how. If not, then explain why.

_____

_____

_____

_____

2: Choose a bro. How often do you initiate a talk, a chat, or a hangout with him?

_____

_____

_____

_____

3: Imagine that one of your bros suddenly stopped taking the initiative to meet you. What would you do? (If it has happened in your life, feel free to use it in your answer.)

_____

_____

_____

_____

4: Is there anything in your life that needs to be prioritized a bit less in order for your friendships to be prioritized more?

_____

_____

_____

_____

5: What season of life are you in? What seasons are your best bros in?

_____

_____

_____

_____

6: Do you think you need to be a bit more intentional or a bit more relaxed and organic in your friendships? Explain your answer.

_____

_____

_____

_____

—

TAKE ACTION

What can you practically do to implement what you've learned in this chapter in your own life?

_____

_____

_____

_____

28: Wounds That Shape Us

We've all got a past, a story. And whether I like to admit it or not, though I don't want my past to dictate my future, I can't ignore the past and the marks it has left on me. I have to acknowledge it to be able to move ahead.

I've experienced some of the best moments of my life in my friendships. But I've also experienced lots of pain as well. When we get close to someone, we allow them to see who we are. We allow ourselves to be vulnerable. We also allow them to get so close that they can touch our wounds from the past. And sometimes that can hurt. Being close is beautiful, but it can also be scary.

If you've experienced abandonment, a broken friendship or relationship, trauma or abuse in your life, don't be surprised if you see some of these wounds come up in your current close friendships. When they do come up, it's important to be honest about it. If you're for example afraid of being left or abandoned by someone you love then being close to someone might create a lot of anxiety. This anxiety will probably affect your behavior, and if you don't address it, it can create a lot of conflicts. Unaddressed wounds will cause unnecessary conflict. Addressed wounds can cause positive change.

Some say that hurt people hurt people. And we're all in the same boat - we are all 'those people'. What's important is how we deal with our pain from the past. I believe the best way to heal the wounds from the past is by not isolating ourselves from each other, but daring to be close again. Consistent, loving, and caring friendships are perfect places for healing and mending. I'm not saying that it's easy, but when you love someone, you'll go far. You'll take the punches that come your way in order for the other person to heal, and the other way. Are you bros only when it's easy, or for the long haul?

I once talked to a counselor who said that: "If we would do friendship better, I would probably lose my job!" Not that counselors aren't important - they are! And sometimes in life, we might need to talk to someone professional about what we struggle with, but don't under-estimate the power of friendship.

If you want to learn more about how our wounds and our past can affect the way we do close relationships, then I suggest checking out the book *Why You Do The Things You Do* by Gary Sibcy and Tim Clinton.

QUESTIONS TO REFLECT ON

1: Do you have any wounds from the past that might affect your friendships? Have you shared it with a bro?

_____

_____

_____

_____

2: Have you experienced being a part of a bro's healing process? Describe.

_____

_____

_____

_____

—

TAKE ACTION

1: Initiate a conversation with a bro where you talk about this chapter.

29: Reliability & Consistency

This part is so simple yet so challenging. It's about being reliable.

If you're reliable, people will trust you. If you're not reliable, they won't. It's about making an appointment and sticking to it. It's about letting our yes be yes and our no be no.

There's nothing more annoying than trying to be friends with a guy who doesn't keep his word, never shows up on time, cancels his plans whenever he feels like it, or just doesn't show up when he's supposed to. This makes it really hard to create a strong bond.

A practical example from my own life is when a bro has called me and I've been busy and told him that I'll call him back later, but I don't. This may happen a few times without anyone really caring about it, but if it becomes a habit, it'll get really annoying for my friend. Whether the reason I don't call him back (all those times) is a legit reason or not, it's still my responsibility to keep my word. If I make commitments I can't keep, then I just shouldn't make them.

Unreliability in a friendship creates insecurity. And insecurity creates distance. Distance weakens the bond.

Calling a bro back when I've told him I will might seem like a small thing. Showing up on time might seem like a small thing. But it's the small habits that often create big consequences. And if you're not reliable with small things, how can you be reliable with more important things?

It's important that we don't use these things against one another or try to figure out the other person's faults and ignoring our own. But it's totally fine to let a bro know if he's not being reliable. How you say it (and maybe when) is key.

I'd like to add one more thing. It kind of goes hand in hand with reliability. It's consistency. It's about not going from hot to cold, yes to no, committed to not committed. I've been in friendships where I just feel so secure because I know where I've got the other person. He's consistent in his way of being, and he's a consistent friend - he doesn't waver back and forth. I've also experienced the opposite, where a bro has been anything but consistent. This has made me both insecure and not really sure about where I've got him. In those situations, it has been easier for me to withdraw, though what I probably should've done is talk about it. Knowing how much inconsistency in a friendship affects me, I've told myself that I'm gonna do everything in my power to make sure that I'm not being an inconsistent friend. Though I fail from time to time, I get back up, ask for forgiveness when necessary, and try to get better.

QUESTIONS TO REFLECT ON

1: Would you consider yourself as a reliable bro? In what ways?

_____

_____

_____

_____

_____

2: Are there any areas in your friendship life where you could be more reliable (letting your yes be yes and no be no)?

_____

_____

_____

_____

3: How does it make you feel when a bro is inconsistent? Does it encourage you to get closer to him or the opposite? Describe a situation where you've experienced inconsistency.

_____

_____

_____

_____

4: Choose a bro. In what ways is he reliable and consistent?

_____

_____

_____

_____

—

TAKE ACTION

What can you practically do to implement what you've learned in this chapter in your own life?

_____

_____

_____

_____

30: Cheap Excuses Are Worthless

Cheap excuses are never cool. If I've got a reliability issue, a relational issue, or any other character issue for that matter, I need to own it and not come up with excuses not to do anything about it. Being aware of our own flaws is important because whether you like it or not, these flaws will affect your friendships.

If you ever meet a dude who tells you: "Just a heads up, I really suck at staying in touch with my friends. Just so you know," then you've most likely met a person whom it'll be difficult to create a consistent and solid friendship with. Not because he's got issues (we all have), but because his excuse suggests that he's not making any active effort to change.

Some say that their character issue is a part of who they are and that they can't change who they are. Well… I simply can't say that "it's my personality not to be reliable or committed," and if I do, it's just a clear sign that I'm avoiding taking responsibility for my own life and my relationships. It's childish to use our 'personality' as an excuse not to improve as a person or as a friend. Excuses are easy to come up with, but they take us nowhere.

QUESTIONS TO REFLECT ON

1: Are there any 'personality traits' - or other things in your life, that you might use as an excuse not to grow as a friend?

_____

_____

_____

_____

2: Based on your answer to question 1, what do you want to do about it?

_____

_____

_____

_____

31: Empowering Others

A good friendship should empower others. If I become a worse version of myself when hanging out with a friend, then I should talk to my friend about it and try to change it or reflect on whether or not I should keep investing in that friendship.

A good friendship also ought to encourage the ones around you. Have you ever been hanging out with some people, like a couple or a pair of best friends, and you feel like the odd one out? I have, and I'm sure I've made other people feel like the odd one out at times as well. But I don't want any of my relationships (whether with a friend or a girlfriend) to make other people feel excluded. I appreciate quality time with my bros more than anything, but when we surround ourselves with other people, let's make them feel seen and valued.

If a bro and I see a guy at a party who hasn't got anyone to talk to, then we have two choices. We can either choose to ignore him and just enjoy each other's company or we could walk over to him and get to know him. Choosing the latter will result in me and my bro not being able to talk about everything we wanted to talk about that night, but instead, we would get to know someone new, and make a difference in someone else's life. It's a basic example, but you get the idea. The extent to which a friendship thrives will depend on how much of a 'blessing' the friendship is to others. Any relationship that only seeks itself is a waste of time. A relationship that blesses others always wins. You never lose by giving.

I love it when I've had people come up to me and one of my bros and expressed how inspired they are by our friendship. So I've decided that if my closest friendships don't make a positive impact on the people around me, then something's gotta change.

QUESTIONS TO REFLECT ON

1: Choose one of your friendships. To what degree is your brotherhood 'being a blessing' to others?

_____

_____

_____

_____

2: How inclusive are you and your bros with other people?

_____

_____

_____

_____

3: Choose a bro. In what way could you guys be even more outward-focused? (Meaning: together caring for others, making a difference in other people's lives, etc.)

_____

_____

_____

_____

32: Give and Take

A friendship has to go both ways. A friendship that is not built on mutual love, respect and support will sooner or later become dysfunctional.

We give and take, but not necessarily at the same time. Sometimes I've had to give more and receive less, and other times I've given less and received more. I've experienced seasons in life where I've had to lean on a brother's shoulder, and seasons where I've had to be that shoulder for my bro to lean on. If I'm the only one leaning on my bro, though, and never the other way, then it can become a bit unbalanced. If you experience a friendship that only goes one way over an exceedingly long period of time, then it would be smart to talk about it.

We've all got different personalities and we can tend to take the same roles in our social life. I am an initiative taker by nature (if that's even a thing). I tend to be the first one to reach out and start conversations with people I don't know. If I think someone's cool and I'd like to get to know them, I'm not hesitating to invite them out for a coffee. I have also experienced many times that I've taken most of the initiative in some of my friendships and that doesn't automatically mean the friendship is unbalanced. It can simply mean that I've just taken the 'role' as the initiative taker in the friendship. But if I do end up finding it a bit annoying to mostly having to be the one taking initiative, then I should reach out and just talk about it.

A healthy friendship doesn't keep a record of who's done the most. It doesn't even require you to express the same amount of vulnerability (though expressing some is important). A healthy friendship just has to consist of two people who are willing to mutually love and respect one another.

QUESTIONS TO REFLECT ON

1: Have you ever found yourself in a not mutually loving friendship? Describe.

_____

_____

_____

_____

2: Are there any of your friendships that are a little bit unbalanced? What makes it unbalanced and what do you want to do about it?

_____

_____

_____

_____

_____

33: Touch Isolation

Have you ever wondered why it's accepted for girls to express physical affection in their friendships, while it's often frowned upon if we guys do it?

Have you ever felt uncomfortable when giving a bro a hug that has been a bit too gentle (instead of the pat on the back) or a hug that has lasted for a bit too long? Have you ever felt like, as a guy, you need to be careful with how much affection you express towards a bro?

Let me introduce you to a topic that I almost didn't want to bring up, because some of you cringe by just hearing the words physical affection and men's friendship in one sentence. But the truth is that physical touch is a part of our humanity. It's a way of communicating, bonding, comforting, and caring for one another. Too many boys and men are living their lives completely touch isolated. And don't think they can do that without facing any consequences - human touch not only calms and comforts us (when we're sad) or makes us feel connected and close (when we hug someone we love). Just do a Google search on the importance of human touch and you'll see that it affects every part of who you are - including your emotional, psychological, and physical health.

Girls can give each other a cuddle. Guys can't. That's gay, apparently. Girls can give each other a gentle hug or look into each others' eyes while saying "I love you". Guys can't. That's gay, apparently. Girls can express lots of joy when seeing one another. Guys can't. That's gay, apparently. And it goes on.

We live in a world where men's actions have been sexualized big time. As a result, many men avoid any physical contact, especially with their guy friends, in order for it to not be perceived as sexual. To some of us, being close to another guy, or expressing gentleness towards another guy, simply feels wrong. It feels awkward and unnatural. A toddler, though, freely expresses love for whoever is around him. A man freaks out. What's wrong here? Are men really created to live lives without any platonic touch? No wonder why many guys are desperate for sex. As mentioned earlier, they go to the club, they find someone, hook up and end up in bed. Their desire for physical touch and gentleness conflates with their sexual desires, leading to a cheap and fake intimacy.

As a man myself, I've experienced that it's more accepted to express physical touch in my male friendships as long as I'm not being too gentle. I need to add a little bit of roughness, or I at least need to make sure the physical contact doesn't last for too long. I can also be physically close if I have an excuse to be. For example, if we're working out, I can help my gym buddy finish his last pull-ups. Another way to be physical is to joke about it, like the teenage boys who when hugging or touching a bro gently, laughs, and calls each other gay. Deep down, they're actually craving that touch they're taught to reject and make fun of.

In my own life, I've found myself hesitating on either giving or receiving affection from a bro, not really knowing if my bro thinks it's okay to be close, if I myself think it is okay, or if others do. It's happened more than once that a friend and I have hugged and someone has shouted "gay" at us. It's also happened more than once that a bro and I have expressed affection for each other, and someone has commented: "Guys, you both need to get yourselves a girlfriend..." My questions is: How often do you hear people say that to girls when they are physically close: "Hey girls. You need to get yourselves a boyfriend."

You might feel really uncomfortable reading about this topic, you might not. But the more uncomfortable you are, the more of a taboo it probably is to you. And changing it doesn't happen overnight. The mindset that 'guys shouldn't express physical affection towards guys' has to many of us become the norm. And as a result, our brain and our body now rejects even the idea of being physically close to another man.

Also. Have you ever wondered why it's fine for male athletes to hug and be physical during a rugby match, for example, but not for the average guy on the street? Here's my answer: They're 'allowed' to express themselves like this because they're already doing something that is considered masculine. They can hug, kiss, or slap a teammate's butt after scoring a goal without their masculinity or heterosexuality being questioned. Being an athlete (doing something 'masculine') works as a cover for them to express themselves in ways that otherwise would've labeled them gay. It's also the same with guys with a high social status. Their status actually gives them more freedom to express, in this instance, affection towards their mates, without being questioned.

Male friendships do look more or less different in different cultures and what we might perceive as normal behavior for guys in their friendships in one country might not be considered normal in another country. I talked to a couple of guys who'd been in India, and at first, they thought there were so many gay dudes there - until they were told that it was normal for guy friends to hold hands there - just like many female friends hold hands in the Western world. But again - what's culturally accepted in one city, might not be culturally accepted in another city - even though in the same country. You can even say the same about individuals. Even though I've lived in Western countries my whole life (Norway and Australia), I've encountered guys who literally cringe at the thought of giving their best bro a warm hug - to meeting guys who're way more affectionate in their friendships than most girls that I've met.

But know this - my goal is not to make guys cuddle more. My goal is to see you be able to freely give and receive platonic touch from your mates. Appreciating physical touch is not weird or unnatural - it's healthy.

I'm well aware of the fact that not everyone is a physical touch kind of person in general, and that we all express love in different ways, but if you find it uncomfortable to hug a guy, but not a girl, then I urge you to do some reflecting and figure out why.

And though I've been writing about the importance of gentle touch, I'm not saying that a handshake, a pat on the back, a wrestle or anything that is 'rough' isn't good. I'm the kinda guy who thinks it's cool messing around, cracking jokes with my boys, slapping them in the stomach, being cheeky, wrestling, and all that. But I also appreciate getting an arm around my shoulder or a warm hug that lasts for more than a second from a bro. My desire is for us to freely express our love for each other, without having the stigma hinder us from it.

PS. If you found what I've written so far about this topic uncomfortable, the reflections will be even more confronting. Just a heads up.

QUESTIONS TO REFLECT ON

1: Have you refrained from physical closeness in a friendship with a guy? If yes, then why?

_____

_____

_____

_____

2: What would your reaction be if your best bro asked you for a hug?

_____

_____

_____

_____

3: Would you find it easier to express affection towards a girl than towards your best guy friend? Explain why/why not.

_____

_____

_____

_____

4: Imagine two girls being affectionate. What would you assume? Then two guys. What would you assume? Explain why.

_____

_____

_____

_____

5: How much do you value platonic touch in your own friend-ships? Is it a part of your friendships?

_____

_____

_____

_____

6: Humans use physical touch to communicate. Write down different ways you use touch in order to communicate with your bros.

_____

_____

_____

_____

7: Remove *all* physical touch between you and your bros. How do you think it would affect your friendship?

_____

_____

_____

8: How comfortable are you with expressing gentle physical touch towards a bro versus rough or aggressive physical touch towards a bro?

_____

_____

_____

_____

9: If you're an athlete, then write down different ways you use physical touch during a match. Now remove all physical touch between you and your teammates - how do you think this would affect your performance and your team?

_____

_____

_____

_____

—

TAKE ACTION

1: Initiate a conversation about this topic with a bro.

34: Every Brotherhood is Different

Throughout life, we'll have many different friendships. Most of them will be for seasons, some of them will be for life. We will have best friends, close friends, good friends, general friends, and acquaintances. As a super extroverted guy, I've got lots of general friends, many good friends, a few close friends, and less than a handful of best friends.

My best mates are the ones I invest in on a frequent and regular basis, but I also really value the connections I've got with the boys who I see less often. I've also got some bros who come and go in my life and though they've only been in my life for a short season, they've made a huge impact on my life.

The Real Bro Code is focusing mostly on our closest friendships, but it's important to value the different kinds of friendships that we have. I know many guys who are just awesome, super entertaining, adventurous, inspiring, and full of life - but we still only see each other when we bump into each other. I can't say why we don't spend more time together, but I know I can't be best bros and spend lots of time with every guy that I think rocks.

Because all my friends are different and have different personalities and interest, I also have to approach every friendship differently. My friendship with Logan looks different from my friendship with Dan. And my friendship with Dan looks completely different than my friendship with Ben. Don't try to fit all your friendships into the same box; you'll end up suffocating some of them. They will feel forced and unnatural. We must learn to appreciate the uniqueness of each friendship or we'll never be satisfied with any of them.

QUESTIONS TO REFLECT ON

1: Pick two or more of your closest bros. Describe the dynamics of each friendship (e.g., aspects that make it special, things you normally do or talk about, what makes it unique.)

_____

_____

_____

_____

_____

_____

2: How do you differentiate between a best bro versus a good bro?

_____

_____

_____

3: Who are some of the guys you really value but you won't necessarily call them your best bros? Write down what you value about them.

_____

_____

_____

_____

35: Space

In any relationship, it's important to respect each other's need for space. Sometimes I just feel like I wanna be alone or spend some time with someone else – and that doesn't mean that I don't love my bro anymore. It just means I need some space. But it gets tricky when one friend wants space but another wants 'togetherness'. When that happens, one person has to let go of their need, for the sake of the other. Again, we gotta give and take.

If I trust my bro and if I'm secure about our friendship, then I won't freak out if he tells me he needs some space or he doesn't want to hang out one night. It's also nice to be apart from the ones we care about sometimes. It'll give us the chance to miss them.

Our ability to be close and also apart from our closest friends also depends on other factors. You might be someone who've experienced trauma or abandonment in your life, so if a bro (or someone else you love) needs space, you might interpret it as rejection. If this is an issue in your life, then I encourage you to talk to a bro about it. Express your insecurity and say that you want to learn how to be close, but also be apart, without being afraid. If it is a huge problem in your life, then chatting to a counselor can also be an idea.

—

QUESTIONS TO REFLECT ON

1: Describe a time when you've needed space in one of your friendships. How did you communicate it?

_____

_____

_____

_____

2: Describe a time when a bro has expressed that he's needed some space. How did you deal with it?

_____

_____

_____

_____

36: Betrayal

Some friendships end as a result of betrayal. And to be honest, I've both felt betrayed and done the betraying myself. It happens, but it's important to learn how to deal with it.

There are many reasons why betrayal may happen: greed, pride, desire, conflict, selfishness, jealousy, unawareness – just to mention a few. It might also be a result of a person's poor ability to form and sustain close relationships, which again is probably a result of upbringing and past. The stigma around men's friendships doesn't really help to prevent betrayal either.

What breaks my heart is listening to guys (who normally act very cool, laidback or emotionally stoic) express how they feel let down by their friend and how the trust in their relationship has been broken. My best advice when facing disappointments like this is to always forgive and try to reconcile. Instead of ditching your bro straight away, give him another chance. You may appreciate another chance too one day. Too many men just leave their guy friend when they've felt betrayed, without even talking about it.

So have a chat with your friend and tell him how you

feel. If he recognizes his mistake and asks for forgiveness, then good. This experience will hopefully just strengthen your friendship. If he doesn't want to own his mistakes, then it's a bit more difficult. You'll have to figure out if you'd like to continue being his friend and forgive and forget without him acknowledging that he hurt you. I can't figure that out for you; it's your decision.

You might sit there and think that you're the one who betrayed a bro once. If that's the case, then, again: talk about it with your bro if it's possible or appropriate. Whether or not the friendship will be mended, remember to ask for forgiveness regardless.

QUESTIONS TO REFLECT ON

1: Have you ever betrayed a bro before? Why? And what happened after?

_____

_____

_____

_____

_____

2: Have you ever felt betrayed by a bro? How did you deal with it?

_____

_____

_____

_____

_____

37: When A Brotherhood Ends

You might have had a solid friendship, and you've both been committed, authentic, real, and all that good stuff. But still, somehow, the friendship took an end.

Maybe you've lost a close friend in an accident, maybe you've lost a friend because of an argument, betrayal, or maybe you chose to walk different ways. Maybe the friendship simply faded away or maybe you chose to end it. Regardless of how it happens, it happens, and grieving is a natural part when losing someone.

The end of a friendship is often no less painful than the break-up of a dating relationship. For some, it can be worse.

Some of you guys have tried to ignore the pain you've faced after the end of a friendship. You've felt like it's wrong for you to feel a strong sense of loss and sadness, especially since it's caused by another guy and not a girl. Well, I guess it's time to acknowledge that loss and those emotions, and don't think it's unnatural to grieve over the loss of a bro.

When a friendship ends, there are new ones right around the corner. Just remember to leave on good terms (if possible), appreciate the time you had together, and learn from your mistakes.

—

QUESTIONS TO REFLECT ON

1: Have you ever lost a bro? Why? And how did you deal with it?

_____

_____

_____

_____

_____

38: Dreams, Goals, & Purpose

Having dreams, goals and a purpose in life will help you get out of bed in the morning. But as a bro, I don't want to be so focused on my own dreams and goals that I totally ignore my friends' dreams and goals.

I want to be my bro's biggest fan and I want to help him succeed and reach his dreams. I want to celebrate his victories and be there with him when he loses. I want to remind him of his purpose when he doesn't see it himself and help him reach the finish line when he doesn't have enough strength to cross it. Life is much better when we have someone to win together with and fail together with. Don't let your bro win or fail alone.

I wanna be my bro's biggest fan because I know I need a bro like that myself. Someone who cares about my dreams and my goals, not just his own.

If it wouldn't have been for my mates being willing to sacrifice time and energy to help me, Brothers wouldn't have been the movement that it is today and you wouldn't have held The Real Bro Code in your hands.

QUESTIONS TO REFLECT ON

1: Choose two bros. What are some of their dreams and goals?

_____

_____

_____

_____

2: How can you help them accomplish these dreams and goals?

_____

_____

_____

_____

3: Describe a situation where you've celebrated one of your bros' victories.

_____

_____

_____

_____

4: Describe a moment where either you've almost given up on something in life, or a bro has, but because you encouraged each other and were there for one another, you didn't give up.

_____

5: To what degree do you feel like your friendships are pur-pose-filled?

_____

—

TAKE ACTION

1: Ask a bro what some of his dreams are and ask him what you can do to help him reach them.

39: Upbringing

We're all more or less shaped by our surroundings. What type of family you grow up in will to some degree affect the way you behave and think.

A guy I know, Luke, comes from a pretty closed-off family. He told me that they don't normally talk about how they feel or anything like that. I asked him in what way that had affected his friendships and he said: "I think it has affected my friendships quite a lot. I find it hard to talk about how I feel with anyone, to be honest. Growing up I was never used to it."

After talking a bit more with Luke, I realized that his family life wasn't uncomplicated. Though he, of course, had lots of good memories with his family, he told me that he didn't have a really good relationship with his father. When Luke was a kid, his dad wasn't very present in his life. As for any kid, having a distant father is painful, and it took years for Luke before he started dealing with this pain. A father really has a lot to say in his child's identity development, something that is of great importance in a time and age where so many boys and grown-up men have no clue about who they are.

I've heard *many* stories of guys not having a good connection with their dad. Not surprisingly, the same guys also don't recall their dad having deep friendships. This leaves their sons with no solid reference to what a deep male friendship can look like. And if their dad won't show them how to bond with other men, then who will?

—

QUESTIONS TO REFLECT ON

1: How would you say your family upbringing has shaped your way of doing friendship with your boys?

_____

_____

_____

_____

_____

2: What does/did your dad's friendships look like?

_____

_____

_____

_____

_____

3: What does/did your mom's friendships look like?

_____

_____

_____

_____

4: Choose a bro. How do you think his family upbringing has affected his way of doing friendship?

_____

_____

_____

_____

40: Investment & Generosity

Having a friendship is like an investment. If you value it a lot, you'll invest in it a lot. Some people don't invest in their friendship because they don't value their friendship. And some don't value their friendship because they haven't experienced real friendship.

If you invest nothing into a connection, you'll get nothing out of it. If you invest a lot, you'll reap a lot. We can invest in our friendships with our time, our energy, with words, commitment, compliments, or our money. We simply can't be stingy if we want a solid brotherhood.

Nick, a guy I chatted to, told me this:

> Me and my best bro have this thing where if, for example, he needs to buy something or whatever, he can just ask for my credit card and I'll give it to him without asking what he's gonna used it for and he can just use it. It's pretty nice, actually. And it goes both ways. What is mine is his and I trust him.

I actually really like that! And though generosity should be and can be expressed through more than just money, our bank account gives us a pretty good insight into what we care about the most. My goal is to become more and more generous with my time, energy, compliments, money, and everything that I have. I wanna be generous with my bros and honestly, with everyone that I meet.

—

QUESTIONS TO REFLECT ON

1: In what ways are you practically investing in your friendships?

_____

_____

_____

_____

2: In what ways can you be more generous in your friendships? (e.g., with compliments, money, energy, time.)

_____

_____

_____

_____

TAKE ACTION

1: Come up with a way you can practically extend generosity towards a bro in the next week. Whether it is by filling up his car one day, paying for his dinner, helping him move, helping him clean his apartment, or whatever.

41: Bro-Dating

Take good care of the bros you've already got but be open to new friendships as well. Different people enrich our lives and bring out sides in us that otherwise would've been hidden.

Sometimes in life, I've gotten an instant connection with some guys. We've both experienced a 'high' or excitement when meeting each other and it's rad; it's like a kick-starter to a new friendship. Though some guys don't want to admit it, experiencing chemistry with a bro is normal. It's almost like a 'bro crush'…

Anyway. Sometimes you'll experience some real bro-mance. Other times a friendship doesn't seem too exciting in the beginning, but when you give it a shot, and when you get to know the other guy, a solid friendship might start taking form. I've also met guys whom I haven't really connected with at all in the beginning, but after a little while they've grown on me and suddenly we've become really close.

Sometimes I've had to be really intentional when approaching a dude, and I've had to express my interested in getting to know him - other times we've just ended up becoming mates quite randomly.

All this to say that there is not a set way on how a friendship should start. We just gotta throw ourselves into it.

New friendships are cool. We spend time with each other, and hopefully, at some point, we evaluate whether we'd like to pursue a deeper connection. Is this best-bro material, or just a good, but casual friendship? You might think this process sounds a bit like dating... Well, I call it bro-dating. It's important to choose your friends wisely. But remember to not write off a friendship before you've gotten to know each other. Maybe you'll end up being super close. Maybe not. Time will show.

When a friendship is new, it's good to be both intentional and let it flow its natural course. As a guy who thinks a lot, I've found myself overthinking quite often. In the process of figuring out 'where I've got him', whether or not I find him trustable and reliable, for example, I've had to remind myself that building a friendship takes time, and that sometimes I gotta chill out and drop all expectations and see where it ends up. And you won't know after just a few hangouts if this is a bro to your destiny or not.

QUESTIONS TO REFLECT ON

1: Any 'bro-dating' going on in your life at the moment?

_____

_____

_____

_____

2: Choose a bro. How did your friendship start?

_____

_____

_____

_____

_____

3: Choose another bro. How did your friendship start?

_____

_____

_____

_____

_____

42: Everyday Life of Brotherhood

The Real Bro Code hopefully inspires you to not settle for mediocrity in your guy friendships. But I also want to remind you not to be afraid of the everyday life of brotherhood.

I appreciate adventure and adrenaline. For me, living in a big city, I'm constantly exposed to crowds, entertainment, and stuff to do. But I also know how crucial it is for me not to expect my friendships with my bros to be hyped or full of adventure all the time. There will be boring times and everyday, normal days in any relationship, and that's okay. My ability to enjoy these mundane times in my friendships will determine how long my friendships will last.

What I appreciate the most about my closest bros is to be able to be quiet together and hang out without having an agenda. A friendship where you have to be full of energy and always be 'on' will make you exhausted after a time. Not that I don't enjoy being crazy. I'm a sicko myself and can go nuts with the boys. But there's a time for everything.

Like anything good in life, we can easily take it for granted when we've been exposed to it for long enough, and our deepest connections are no different. Like the new car that we got. It was so cool in the beginning, but then we got familiar with it and now we don't really appreciate it anymore. Or that school that we got accepted into. At first, we were stoked that we got in, but after a little while, we got so used to it and even started complaining about the very thing that we at first really wanted.

It's vital that we don't let over-familiarity tear on the connection we have with our closest mates. I've found myself sometimes taking a bro for granted. Maybe we've been mates for a few years, and the very things that I appreciated about him in the beginning, I don't really care about anymore. People say you don't really know how much someone means to you until you lose them. Well, don't wait for you to lose your bro until you value him.

QUESTIONS TO REFLECT ON

1: How comfortable are you with being quiet with your bros?

_____

_____

_____

_____

2: Any friendships or qualities in a bro that you've taken for granted lately?

_____

_____

_____

_____

43: How to Find Bros

You might have been reading through The Real Bro Code, tried to reflect on the questions and tried to do the points of action, but you struggle to think of any friendships you could put into practice what you've learned. For whatever reason, you don't have any bros to go deeper with, go on adventures with, watch a rugby game with or call when you need advice. Truth is that you're not the only one. There are thousands of guys in the same situation. But I've got good news for you: it doesn't have to be like this forever.

The most important thing is to not give up. You might be so sick of trying to reach out but getting nowhere, that you've given up on reaching out anymore. If that's you, then I challenge you to give it another shot. The fear of rejection can sometimes hinder us from approaching new friendships, but if we don't take any chances we won't win. Putting yourself out there is risky, but it's worth it when you find a great connection.

The degree of how difficult it is to find friends often depends on what life situation we find ourselves in. Here's what Will (22) told me:

> I feel like it gets harder to find new friends the older you get. When I was younger I would always be surrounded by people, starting from kindergarten to soccer practice to school to college. (…) Also, when people pass adolescence and become adults, they tend to have found their crew, so to say, and they're not so interested in forming new friendships.

What Will describes here is a common thing. It does tend to get more difficult to form new friendships the older you get. When we pass our mid-twenties, we might not be surrounded by as many people anymore, people have found their circle of friends and we tend to be a bit more suspicious and closed off when meeting new people. The way we prioritize our time and who we spend it with and evaluate whether we should enter into a new friendship or not, looks quite different to when we were thirteen.

When I was thirteen, I just became friends with whoever I met and liked. Now, I think much more about: "is this a friendship worth investing in?" or "is this a guy who's got the same values as me?" or "are we heading in the same direction in life?" Yes, let's not throw those questions out of the window, but let's also not completely forget how easily we would connect with people when we were kids. Though life gets more complex and even more complicated as we get older—with all its responsibilities and challenges—I'm giving a vote for embracing a bit of the childlike, laid-back, and worry-free way of connecting.

Okay, so now I've written about all the challenges. But

how do you actually find friends? Here are some suggestions:

- Position yourself in the right place. (Meaning, don't sit at home watching TV, hoping that someone will knock on your door and ask to be your bro.)

- Take initiative.

- Be open and aware.

- Ask yourself if there are any guys at your school, university, sports club, workplace, in your church or your neighborhood, or anywhere else who you'd like to get to know better. If there are, be bold and reach out to him/them. Ask if they'd like to grab a coffee, a beer, play a sport, or do something fun together.

- If you don't attend any of the activities mentioned above, then start doing it.

It's also nice mentioning that you should be patient. You don't want to be that guy who's so desperate for connection that he tries to BFF someone after one coffee. Though the feeling of loneliness or desperation might be valid, try to take it easy. Sharing your whole life story with a bloke that you don't even know might not always be the best move.

Another advice is to do some self-reflection. If I'm constantly negative and complain about everything - or completely selfish and self-centered, then I probably won't have a line of guys wanting to be my bro either. We all have more or less annoying habits, so dare to ask yourself what attitudes or habits you have that might be pushing people away rather than inviting people to become your friend.

And hey, feeling lonely or not having any close bros is not unusual. I've experienced both loneliness and the lack of friendship in my own life, and it sucks. Really. But know that you're not alone. What you've got to do is acknowledge where you're at and then do something about it. Just don't give up.

So put yourself out there and have one goal: Make sure that the people you meet leave feeling better about themselves than when they first met you. Continue doing that and I'm pretty sure you'll end up with some cool bro-connections.

You can do it.

QUESTIONS TO REFLECT ON

1: How do you connect with new people now versus when you were ten years old?

_____

_____

_____

2: To what degree do you find it hard/easy to find new bros?

_____

_____

_____

3: Are there any attitudes or habits you have that might be pushing people away rather than inviting them to create a friendship? If yes, then how can you change this?

_____

_____

_____

4: Are you open to new friendships in your life? And when was the last time you got to know a new dude?

_____

_____

_____

TAKE ACTION

1: If you need friends, write down a list of possible guys you can catch up with. Make sure that within a week, you've gotten in touch with at least some of them and planned a catch-up.

2: If you can't think of anyone, then write down a few suggestions/places where you could meet people. Write down when you will go there and how often. You gotta put yourself out there.

3: Sit down and write down more ideas on how to find friends.

4: If you know a guy who struggles to find friends, then help him out. Let him know about The Real Bro Code. You might not be able to be his best bro yourself, but you might be able to help him in the right direction.

5: If you tend to be too closed off to new guys, maybe approach a dude you'd like to get to know a bit more and invite him out for a beer or something.

44: Self-Reflection

I'd like to invite you to do some self-reflection. As a part of the self-reflection, I advise you to celebrate your strengths as a bro and write down practical ways to improve.

—

QUESTIONS TO REFLECT ON

1: What parts of The Real Bro Code did you find the most challenging? And why?

_____

_____

_____

_____

_____

2: What are some of the qualities you think your bros appreciate about you the most?

_____

_____

_____

3: What do you wanna get better at as a bro? Go through the different chapters if you need a refresher.

_____

_____

_____

_____

4: Based on your answer to questions 3, what are some practical steps you can take to improve on these things?

_____

_____

_____

_____

5: Choose one or two of your friendships. After reading The Real Bro Code, in what ways would you like your friendship with each of these guys to grow?

_____

_____

_____

_____

6: Based on your answer to questions 5, what are some practical things you can do together as bros, to make this happen?

_____

_____

_____

_____

—

TAKE ACTION

1: Reflect on the questions in the different chapters in The Real Bro Code *with a bro*. It'll without a doubt create some cool and helpful conversations that will encourage you both!

2: Ask a bro for feedback. How can you improve as a friend?

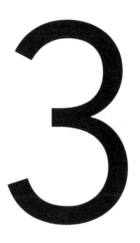

PART THREE
THE OUTRO

BROTHERS
BROTHERS
BROTHERS
BROTHERS
BROTHERS
BROTHERS

Bro! Good job! You've completed part 2! I trust that you've spent more time reflecting and writing down your answers than you've been reading. If you've been really honest and if you have reflected well, then you probably don't wanna lose this book or your notes in case someone else reads it. If you somehow haven't done the questions, then please go back and do it as you've missed out on at least half of the book.

Let's remember again that there's no formula for relationships. People are organic and ever-changing, and our relationships are no different. Though being intentional and practical is good, it will make a friendship unnatural and mechanical if you focus only on that. There's a time to be intentional and a time to just let it flow its natural course. Human relationships are so complex and beautiful, and it takes more than a lifetime to figure them out. I hope, though, that The Real Bro Code has helped you on the way, and that you've been challenged, inspired, and provoked to thought and stirred to take action based on what you've learned and reflected upon. And even though there are hundreds of more topics I could've written about I think it's good that we started with only a few.

The Real Bro Code's goal is not to narrow down our perception of male friendship, but rather to broaden it. As you've been invited to evaluate and reflect intensely on the topic of friendship and your own friendships, it's time to live it out. Maybe the gap between the ideal and the reality has increased, but it's good to have something to reach for. Remember to enjoy the journey.

I hope that those of you who've found it hard to be either close, authentic, vulnerable, or express affection in your guy friendships, have started to embrace what you previously regarded as awkward or not 'manly enough'. Close brotherhood is for all dudes. Every guy needs a bro.

You might be one of those who've realized that your friendships aren't as deep as you thought. If that's you, then stay calm and know that if the willingness is there, it can only get better.

Or you might be that guy who's just rockin' being a bro, and you value your mates more than words can explain. Well aware of the fact that you're not perfect, you've allowed The Real Bro Code to put more fuel on the fire - so that you can continue to grow your connections with the boys you care about.

My hope is also that the guys who've given up on friendship a long time ago - will start to believe in friendship again.

If you're a leader in any way or form (e.g. a teacher, politician, sports coach, CEO) or if you've got a massive sphere of influence (if you're an athlete, celebrity, influencer etc.) then remember that your perception and view of male bonding affects the boys/men you lead and influence, and their perception and view of it - which again affects their performance and life quality. If you've got a solid and healthy view of male friendship, then that's good. If you don't, then it's time to alter it. With much influence comes much responsibility.

Okay. So before I let you go, there are a few things I'd like to end with. Number one: don't compare your friendships to others. I might look at Instagram and think that some dudes are having much cooler friendships than what I have, and they go out on much cooler adventures than what me and my bros do. But comparing my ordinary life to someone else's highlights is never a smart move. I gotta value the unique friendships I've got and where they're at right now.

Number two: we're not each other's bros because we can get something out of each other. We're bros because we love each other.

Number three: let's have friendships where it's easy to be authentic, where it's okay to have a bad day, where laughter comes easy, where it's fine to vent and where we celebrate each other's wins. Let love be at the core, dare to trust each other deeply, be quick to forgive and even quicker to ask for forgiveness.

As the founder of the Brothers organization, and as a researcher on male bonding, I've realized that the more and more I learn about friendship, and wrestle with it, the more I have to admit that I don't know a whole lot. Though I often can feel the pressure of people (and myself) expecting me to be a 'bro guru' or the perfect bro, I am quickly reminded that I am far from perfect. Sometimes I hurt my bros. Sometimes I'm insecure. Sometimes I get jealous. Sometimes I'm selfish. Sometimes I do the opposite of what I might be recommending in this book. But one thing I know: whenever I mess up, admitting it to my bro is the best remedy. I have to swallow my pride and admit that I don't always know how to do friendship well. But I am doing my best - because my friendships with my guys mean ridiculously much to me.

True brotherhood... There's nothing quite like it.

GET YOUR BROS ON BOARD

So. Do you believe that there is more in your friendships? More potential, more fun, more depth, more adventure, and more purpose?

Well, that's awesome! But like any relationship, a friendship involves two people, and in order to move forward, you gotta move forward together.

My passion is to see your friendships go from strength to strength. As you invite your bros on this journey, remember to be patient with each other as you move forward. Change doesn't happen overnight.

I've encouraged you to pursue the fullness of friendship. That means that some of you might have to raise the bar a bit and expect a bit more of yourself (as a bro) and of your friendships. That's not a bad thing. Sometimes we think that having no expectations is a good thing, but that's not necessarily true. If you have no standards in your friendships, you won't care if the friendship is shallow, for example.

But again, that doesn't mean that you should go nuts with your 'new standards'. If you've got a bro who's not used to having deep conversations, for example, don't just throw him into the deep water straight away. Introduce him to Brothers or The Real Bro Code, let him get used to this perspective of male bonding and brotherhood. Give yourself and your bros time to practice and show each other lots of grace when you fall. Reflect on the questions in The Real Bro Code together, and always keep an open line of communication.

You also gotta accept the fact that you will, from time to time, fail and disappoint each other. If you can't handle failure, then stay away from deep friendship. Friendship is a journey, not a destination.

You've finished The Real Bro Code. Or may I suggest that you've just started? Now's the time to put it into practice. And remember: no excuses - they don't help. *Your* friendships are *your* responsibility. Be the bro you want to have in your life yourself. Don't settle for less. Make sure that you don't stop here - make sure the friendship topic is brought up often in your everyday life. If necessary, read The Real Bro Code again. Talk about it with your bros and sisters, family, and co-workers. Just don't do nothing, 'cuz then in a couple of weeks, you'll have forgotten it all.

Your bros are valuable. And so are you. A bro is not just a wingman, a casual hang-out, or a drinking buddy. Look after each other and dare to go above and beyond to care for one another. You never know when it's too late, so don't wait for it to be.

As you embark on the journey ahead of you, remember that I'm cheering for you. And so is Brothers.

And hey. If you haven't already, remember to share The Real Bro Code with your bros. Maybe you can get each of your bros a copy as a gift! I'm sure they'd appreciate it.

If you've got any questions or if you wanna share something with me or the Brothers team, please don't hesitate on reaching out.

And last but not least, thanks to all the ladies out there who believe in and support our work. You rock!

Take care, and thank you for reading The Real Bro Code!

BROTHERS ON ONLINE PLATFORMS

Instagram: @wearebrothersorg

Facebook: facebook.com/wearebrothers.org

Website: wearebrothers.org

Join the movement: wearebrothers.org/join

For booking: contact@wearebrothers.org

BULK ORDERS

The Real Bro Code (the paperback) may be purchased in bulk for educational, business or fundraising use. For information, please e-mail orders@wearebrothers.org

About the Author

Kim is the founder and CEO of Brothers. He has previously studied leadership. After he started the Brothers organization, he has emerged as a subject matter expert on male friendships. He now consults internationally, providing research and presentations about the importance of male friendships and the positive effects arising from strong male relationships. Kim published his first book in 2019, and The Real Bro Code is the second book he's written.

About Brothers

Brothers is a global not-for-profit organization dedicated to empowering men's friendships. Our passion is to see boys and men all over the globe discover what a friendship is and enjoy it to the fullest. Through our sphere of influence, we want to create awareness around the importance of male bonding, offer inspiration and education, and fight any stigma attached to the topic.

Sources and Resources

Books:

"Deep Secrets" by Niobe Way

"Breaking the Male Code" by Robert Garfield

"When Boys Become Boys" by Judy Y Chu

"The Friendship Factor" by Alan Loy McGinnis

"Safe People" by Dr. Henry Cloud

"Why You Do The Things You Do" by Dr. Tim Clinton & Dr. Gary Sibcy

"How to be a Best Friend Forever" by John Townsend

"Dude, You're a Fag" by C. J. Pascoe

"Remaking Manhood" by Mark Greene

"Masculinities" by R. W. Connell

"The Gender of Desire" by Michael Kimmel

"The Crisis of Connection" by Niobe Way, Alisha Ali, Carol Gilligan, and Pedro Noguera

"Brothers: Every Man Needs Strong, Authentic Friendships" by Kim Evensen

Recommended Videos:

"The Mask You Live In" (Documentary)

"Why 'Boys Will Be Boys 'Is A Myth - and a harmful one at that'" (TEDMed talk by Dr. Niobe Way)

+ Interviews for research purposes done by Kim Evensen.

well done, bro

bro – bruh – brah
brother – brotha – pizza

BROTHERS
BROTHERS
BROTHERS
BROTHERS
BROTHERS
BROTHERS

BROTHERS
BROTHERS
BROTHERS
BROTHERS
BROTHERS
BROTHERS

CPSIA information can be obtained
at www.ICGtesting.com
Printed in the USA
LVHW040859181222
735461LV00009B/984